The Official Guide for
Foreign-Educated Nurses

Barbara L. Nichols, DHL, MS, RN, FAAN, is the chief executive officer of CGFNS International (Commission on Graduates of Foreign Nursing Schools), which is an internationally recognized authority on credentials evaluation and verification pertaining to the education, registration, and licensure of nurses and health care professionals worldwide. Ms. Nichols served as professor of nursing at the University of Wisconsin School of Nursing and director of nursing for the Wisconsin Area Health Education Center System. Currently, she serves on the Board of Directors for the American National Standards Institute (ANSI) and is on their Conformity Assessment Policy Committee. She held a cabinet position in Wisconsin State Government, is a former International Council of Nurses (ICN) Board Member and a past President of the American Nurses Association. As Secretary of the Department of Regulation and Licensing for the state of Wisconsin, she was responsible for 17 Boards that regulated 59 occupations and professions. Ms. Nichols is the author of over 70 publications on nursing and health care delivery, including her most recent contribution as a Guest Editor, "Policy, Politics and Nursing Practice," in the August 2006 edition of *Building Global Alliances III: The Impact of Global Nurse Migration on Health Service Delivery.* She was a Lieutenant in the United Sates Navy Nurse Corps. Ms. Nichols was a 2006 Inaugural Inductee into the National Black Nurses Association Institute of Excellence; was named the 2007 Distinguished Scholar, Howard University College of Pharmacy, Nursing and Allied Health Sciences, Division of Nursing; and is a Fellow in the American Academy of Nursing.

Catherine R. Davis, PhD, RN, is the Director of Global Research and Test Administration for CGFNS International. Dr. Davis provides senior leadership for CGFNS test development activities, research initiatives, and related publications. Prior to joining CGFNS International, Dr. Davis was Associate Professor of Nursing at Hahnemann University in Philadelphia. She holds a PhD in Nursing from Adelphi University and a Master's degree in Child and Adolescent Psychiatric Nursing from the University of Pennsylvania. She serves on the National Editorial Advisory Board of Advance for Nurses and as a manuscript reviewer for Sigma Theta Tau International's *Journal of Nursing Scholarship*. Dr. Davis has authored and edited numerous publications on international nursing issues and has served as a national and international speaker on nurse migration trends and challenges, international testing and test development issues, and conducting certification programs.

The Official Guide for Foreign-Educated Nurses

What You Need to Know About Nursing and Health Care in the United States

CGFNS International, Inc.
(Commission on Graduates of Foreign Nursing Schools)

BARBARA L. NICHOLS, DHL, MS, RN, FAAN
CATHERINE R. DAVIS, PHD, RN
EDITORS

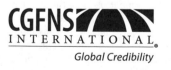

CGFNS
INTERNATIONAL.
Global Credibility

SPRINGER PUBLISHING COMPANY
NEW YORK

Springer Publishing Company, LLC
11 West 42nd Street
New York, NY 10036
www.springerpub.com

Acquisitions Editor: Margaret Zuccarini
Project Manager: Julia Rosen
Cover design: Steve Pisano
Composition: Apex CoVantage, LLC

Ebook ISBN:

09 10 11 / 5 4 3 2 1

Library of Congress Cataloging-in-Publication Data

The official guide for foreign-educated nurses : what you need to know about nursing and health care in the United States / CGFNS International, Inc. (Commission on Graduates of Foreign Nursing Schools) ; Barbara L. Nichols, Catherine R. Davis, editors.
      p. ; cm.
    Includes bibliographical references and index.
    ISBN 978-0-8261-1065-7 (alk. paper)
  1. Nurses, Foreign—United States.   2. Nursing—United States.   I. Nichols, Barbara L.
II. Davis, Catherine R.   III. Commission on Graduates of Foreign Nursing Schools (U.S.)
    [DNLM: 1. Nursing—United States.   2. Delivery of Health Care—United States.
3. Emigration and Immigration—United States. WY 300 AA1 O32 2009]
    RT4.O44 2009
    362.17'3—dc22   2009012551

Printed in the United States of America by Hamilton Printing.

*To all foreign-educated nurses whose wisdom,
courage, and caring spirit give voice and
meaning to the nursing profession worldwide*

Contents

Contributors

Virginia C. Alinsao, MBA, MS, RN, has over 30 years experience in health care and was the Director of International Recruitment for The Johns Hopkins Health System in Baltimore, Maryland. Ms. Alinsao has been an active advocate in the ethical recruitment of international nurses and in supporting transition programs to ensure success of foreign-educated nurses in the United States. She has presented locally and internationally on issues related to international recruitment. As a foreign-educated nurse herself, she will continue advocating in this area.

Winifred Y. Carson-Smith, AB, JD, is founder and chief operating officer of Carson Company, LLC, an advocacy and consulting organization dedicated to changing the paradigm of nursing through policy, regulation, and legislation. Ms. Carson-Smith, former Nursing Practice Counsel for the American Nurses Association, works with clients on health care reform policy, genometrics, informatics, HIV/AIDS policy, drug policy, emergency preparedness, and advanced nurse practice regulation. Ms. Carson-Smith lectures extensively throughout the United States and abroad. She is an author who also publishes the *Nursing Law Report,* an e-newsletter, and the *Nursing Law Alert.* Ms. Carson-Smith is considered an expert on state nursing practice, insurance, and regulatory and administrative law issues. She serves on the editorial advisory boards of the *American Journal of Nurse Practitioners* and *Health Law Week*.

Michael L. Evans, PhD, RN, NEA-BC, FACHE, is the *Maxine Clark and Bob Fox Dean and Professor* at the Goldfarb School of Nursing at Barnes-Jewish College in St. Louis. A chief nurse executive in hospitals for 25 years, his career has bridged hospital and academic nursing administration. His career interests include nursing leadership, workplace enhancement, staff nurse job satisfaction, and workforce innovations.

Lucille A. Joel, EdD, RN, FAAN, is Interim Dean and Professor at Rutgers—the State University of New Jersey College of Nursing, and was Director of the Rutgers Teaching Nursing Home. Dr. Joel has served as President of the American Nurses Association, and the New Jersey State Nurses Association, and as First Vice-president of the International Council of Nurses (ICN), headquartered in Geneva. She currently holds official status as ICN's representative to UNICEF and the United Nations. Dr. Joel is the immediate past-president of the Board of Trustees of CGFNS International.

Marcia M. Rachel, PhD, RN, lives in Brandon, Mississippi, and is the Assistant Dean for Health Systems and Quality Improvement at the University of Mississippi School of Nursing. She was previously the Executive Director of the Mississippi Board of Nursing and also served as Chief Nursing Executive Officer of the University of Mississippi Medical Center. She served as President of the National Council of State Boards of Nursing and is currently President of the Board of Trustees of CGFNS International.

Donna R. Richardson, JD, RN, is the Director of Governmental Affairs and Professional Standards for CGFNS International in Philadelphia, PA. As Director of Governmental Affairs for the American Nurses Association she directed the legislative and regulatory policies that led to the Nursing Immigration Relief Act and occupational health protections for nurses. A registered nurse and attorney she is an experienced lecturer on foreign-educated nurses, minority and women's health issues and clinical trials, and legal issues in nursing and health administration.

Nancy C. Sharts-Hopko, PhD, RN, FAAN, is Professor and Director of the Doctoral Program in the College of Nursing at Villanova University, in Villanova, Pennsylvania. As a veteran of nearly three years working in Asia, first as a short-term consultant for WHO and then as an Overseas Associate of the Presbyterian Church (USA), she understands the challenges associated with living and working in an international context. She has served as an advisory committee member and consultant for the United States Food and Drug Administration since 1992.

Theresa M. "Terry" Valiga, EdD, RN, FAAN, received both her master's and doctoral degree in nursing education from Teachers College, Columbia University in New York. She held faculty and administrative positions in five different universities over a 26-year period, and served as the Chief Program Officer for the National League for Nursing. In July 2008, Dr. Valiga joined Duke University's School of Nursing (Durham, NC) to create and direct their new Institute for Educational Excellence. She has received several awards for excellence in nursing education, and consulted with nursing faculty groups in the United States, Canada, Japan, and China.

Foreword

Nurses migrate to the United States for many reasons. First, nurses in the United States are among the highest paid in the world. Many migrating nurses come to make a better living and, in many cases, share that income with their families back home. Second, U.S. nursing is arguably more complex than nursing in most other countries, in large part due to the pervasive technology for screening, monitoring, and delivering care. Whether the migrating nurse plans to work in acute care, public health, long-term care, or another part of the U.S. health care system, the experience gained in the United States will prepare the nurse with clinical and leadership skills that can be invaluable. Third, some nurses come to the United States to acquire graduate degrees in nursing. Nursing education in the United States is among the most progressive in the world, and there are many opportunities for furthering one's education and qualifications for advanced positions here and abroad. Finally, some nurses may come to the United States for the experience of living in another country. Travel nursing is popular within the United States among nurses who want to see other parts of the country and interact with other cultures—and there are many different cultures within the various geographic regions of the United States. Many of the companies that have specialized in travel nursing within the United States have been expanding their business to other countries, providing another vehicle for nurses to migrate to the United States for work.

Regardless of why you want to work as a nurse in the United States, your entry and transition to working here will be smoother and your contributions more significant if you are knowledgeable about how the health care system functions, what is expected of nurses, what your rights are, how to prepare for the journey, and how to adapt to your new community. No one is better suited to advise you about these matters than Barbara Nichols and Catherine Davis, both with the Commission on Graduates of Foreign Nursing Schools (CGFNS) International, Inc., an internationally-respected, nonprofit organization that evaluates the credentials of health care workers seeking employment in the United States. They have prepared this essential book, *The Official Guide for Foreign-Educated Nurses: What You Need to Know About Nursing and Health Care in the United States,* which will serve as your guide before and after you come to the United States. This book is a "must-read" for every nurse who is contemplating migrating to the United States. I know of no better resource for you, even if you're not yet certain that you want to go to the United States. The guide may help you to make that decision and can assist you in ensuring that you're coming on contractual terms that are clear and beneficial to you.

Once you're in the United States, the book can help you to understand the U.S. health care system and your rights and roles within that system. It can help you determine if your experiences are normal or contrary to the rules that apply to everyone, and it can guide you in your work with U.S. nurses, patients, and families. The book also can help you to figure out ways to avoid being misunderstood in your communication with others and how to increase the likelihood that you'll form enduring relationships with your American colleagues, joining them in working to improve the quality of nursing and health care provided in this country—and worldwide.

I hope that your experience working as a nurse in the United States will be a rich and rewarding one. This nation is often imperfect, as all are, and because of that, it can be an exciting, confusing, joyous, and complicated place to be. While some may assume that you will be the beneficiary of migrating to the United States, I expect that those whom you meet and care for will benefit even more. I have worked with many nurses who migrated to this country and have usually been impressed with their commitment to excellence in nursing, their intellect, and their compassion. Immigrant nurses have become leaders in U.S. nursing and have helped to shape the profession and health care worldwide. During a time of a nursing shortage in the United States, your contributions will help to meet the health care needs of the nation.

Of course, that shortage is worldwide, and there have been many conversations, debates, and arguments about whether nurse migration serves nations well. As the International Council of Nurses (ICN) has argued, migration must be a right for all nurses (read the ICN position statement on the ethical recruitment of nurses in Appendix C or on the ICN Web site at http://www.icn.ch/psrecruit01.htm). At the same time, we must be mindful of the extent to which developed nations are depleting developing or underdeveloped nations of one of their most precious resources—nurses. How can nations such as the United States pay back poorer nations to equalize this shift in resources? You can help to answer this question—whether through sharing your income with your family back home, finding other ways to support the education of nurses in your country, or simply discussing your ideas on this important issue with nurses and others here and abroad.

Our world needs nurses who will be fearless in their commitment to promoting the health of individuals, families, communities, and nations. I urge you to use this book to guide your professional life in the United States, a life that is filled with a sense of responsibility to yourself, your country, the United States, and excellence in nursing. Whether my country or yours, we need your leadership and contributions to the profession and health care.

May your journey to, and within, the United States be resoundingly satisfying, exciting, and enriching. And if our paths happen to cross, please do tell me about your journey.

Diana J. Mason, PhD, RN, FAAN
New York City

Preface

When the Commission on Graduates of Foreign Nursing Schools (CGFNS) International was created in 1977, I was a member of the American Nurses Association Board of Directors and party to the many debates on the efficacy of recruiting foreign nurses to provide patient care to the U.S. population. I was intrigued with the discussion about the advantages and disadvantages of foreign-educated nurses being a temporary or permanent element of the U.S. nursing workforce. What evolved from those discussions was the need to create a program of credentials evaluation that was professionally ethical and responsible to both the foreign-educated nurse and the U.S. public.

The need for an entity such as CGFNS was a novel, yet controversial idea—especially for foreign-educated nurses who felt that assessment of their nursing credentials and a pre-immigration exam to test their nursing knowledge was burdensome and unnecessary. Nevertheless, CGFNS was created at the bequest of the U.S. Department of State, the then–Immigration and Naturalization Service (INS), the U.S. Department of Labor (DOL), and the then–U.S. Department of Health, Education, and Welfare (HEW). Then and now, the need for such an organization emerged from the migration of nurses. Now, as then, a rapidly expanding health care industry welcomes foreign-educated nurses to fill vacancies and to provide care to the U.S. populace.

Adele Herwitz, RN, MS, founding Executive Director of CGFNS, who previously served as an Executive of the American Nurses Association and the International Council of Nurses, played a major role in establishing CGFNS's credibility and guiding the organization to achieve its dual mission—protecting the public of the United States while fostering equitable treatment of nurses around the world.

For over 30 years, CGFNS has served as a valuable resource by reviewing and validating the credentials of migrating nurses seeking employment in the United States. We have vigorously fulfilled our mandate from federal and state governments to uphold the educational and professional standards created to protect the well-being of U.S. citizens receiving care from internationally prepared nurses.

The genesis of this book has emerged from CGFNS's years of dialogue with foreign-educated nurses using our services. The global nursing shortage serves as an ongoing context for our work and intensifies our commitment to both the American public and nurses around the world. We are both respectful and proud of our global presence, its import and impact. We understand that many foreign nurses who migrate do so to improve their lives and those of their families. This fact links the moral substance of our work to reality and challenges us to consider what roles we might play to ensure ethical responses to migration practices.

This book is organized into 11 chapters that present information to assist the reader in what to do when coming to the United States to practice nursing. No doubt the contents of the book will be viewed differently among a variety of readers, but hopefully, all will benefit from the perspective presented.

In chapter 1, "Foreign-Educated Nurses in the United States Health Care System," Barbara Nichols, Catherine Davis, and Donna Richardson briefly trace the history of supply and demand of foreign-educated nurses in the U.S. health care system. The focus on immigration laws, policy, and practices that have influenced the migration of nurses to the United States is informative. Key points for successful adaptation to U.S. nursing practice are succinctly described.

In chapter 2, "Preparing to Leave Your Home Country," Catherine Davis and Donna Richardson identify the many reasons that nurses migrate. The factors that make a host country a favorable destination are depicted. Pitfalls to avoid and ways to reduce the risk of abuse and intimidation also are emphasized. The chapter identifies what you should do in your home country once you decide to move to the United States to work.

In chapter 3, "Entry into the United States," Donna Richardson and Catherine Davis explain the visa requirements to work as a nurse in the United States. Tips for successfully navigating the process for obtaining a visa and a VisaScreen® certificate are provided.

Marcia Rachel, in chapter 4, "Entry into the United States Workforce," addresses nursing licensure in the United States, emphasizing that licensure is at the state level. She provides detailed information on the process to obtain a U.S. nursing license, discusses the requirements for state licensure, and describes both the CGFNS and NCLEX® examinations.

In chapter 5, "Employment in the United States," Michael Evans explains the rights and responsibilities of employees and employers. He spells out the fundamental issues for work success across a variety of health care settings.

Nancy Sharts-Hopko, in chapter 6, "The U.S. Health Care System," offers a broad overview of the scope and structure of the U.S. health care system and how individuals access care. She underscores the importance of knowledge of the health care system as a key to success.

In chapter 7, "Nursing Practice in the United States," Winifred Carson-Smith and Barbara Nichols define and describe nursing practice and the laws and standards that govern professional practice in the United States. They provide a framework for understanding the legal and social elements of professional nursing practice.

In chapter 8, "Communicating in the U.S. Health Care System," Catherine Davis and Donna Richardson focus on interpersonal and English language proficiency challenges that many foreign-educated nurses face as they enter practice in the United States. Through their thorough and thoughtful analysis, they explore the meaning and impact of English language proficiency and interpersonal skills on safe nursing care.

Virginia Alinsao, in chapter 9, "Adjusting to a New Community," provides useful information for newly arriving immigrants adjusting to a new community in the United States. She addresses the major concerns about housing, transportation, and personal safety, all factors that must be considered when adapting to a new country and work environment.

In chapter 10, "Continuing Your Education," Theresa Valiga discusses academic and nonacademic educational programs for nurses in the United States. This chapter outlines the types of nursing education programs and the requirements for academic entry and discusses continuing education programs. The author conveys that a spirit of continuous learning is central to adjusting to working and living in the United States.

Lucille Joel, in chapter 11, "Resources at Your Disposal," provides both a philosophical and practical overview of the U.S. culture and nursing as practiced within that environment. She pursues the theme that success in adapting to a new country is, in part, tied to understanding its culture and its people.

The six Appendices supplement the primary content and are summarized as follows: Appendix A focuses on what you will need as you search for a job in the United States. It contains a sample cover letter requesting an interview, a sample résumé, and a sample letter of thanks following an interview.

Appendix B provides selected U.S. government visa information, focusing specifically on the H-1B and other temporary visa categories as well as permanent visas.

Appendix C provides you with some materials that may be helpful as you begin the process of migrating to the United States. It contains the International Council of Nurses (ICN) Position Statement on Ethical Recruitment as well as forms that you might use to track your correspondence and expenses during migration.

Appendix D provides samples of the CGFNS reports that you may need as you seek a U.S. occupational visa and license to practice. It contains copies of the types of Credentials Evaluation Service (CES) Reports required by many of the State Boards of Nursing, sample Pass and Fail letters for the CGFNS Qualifying Exam^{SM}, and an explanation of the Client Need categories used for the CGFNS and NCLEX-RN® examinations.

Appendix E describes the common slang terms, idioms, jargon, and abbreviations you will encounter in the United States and U.S. Nursing Practice.

Appendix F lists educational resources, namely, a select listing of U.S. schools that provide online nursing degrees.

In creating this book, CGFNS has attempted to provide a bridge that will foster a successful transition for those whose journey brings them to the United States to work. We hope as you read the chapters that not only will we answer your questions and inquiries, but also that you will find the book both informative and helpful.

Barbara L. Nichols, CEO, CGFNS International
Spring 2009

Acknowledgments

We thank the authors for not only taking time to prepare the manuscripts but also for their scholarship, diligence, and enthusiasm. We are indebted to each for helping us realize our goal of creating a helpful, readable book.

Special thanks go to Melanie Jones and Amanda Nickerson, whose attention to detail and indefatigable work to meet deadlines made the book possible, to David Keepnews for his professional assistance, and to Donna R. Richardson for her keen eye and continued support.

We thank Springer Publishing Company, especially Margaret Zuccarini, Executive Acquisitions Editor, and Brian O'Connor, Assistant Editor, for the trust and support they provided throughout the development of the book. Their thought-provoking questions and skill with words transformed a manuscript into a book.

Our gratitude is extended to our colleagues who helped with their encouragement and conversations. They include the CGFNS International Board of Trustees, CGFNS administrative, managerial and operational staff, and the nurses who shared their migration journey with us.

Foreign-Educated Nurses in the U.S. Health Care System

1

BARBARA L. NICHOLS
CATHERINE R. DAVIS
DONNA R. RICHARDSON

In This Chapter

U.S. Immigration Patterns

History of Foreign-Educated Nurses in the U.S. Workforce

Transition to Nursing Practice in the United States

Acculturation

Summary

Keywords

Adjudicate: To settle a case by lawful procedure.

Codified: Signifies that laws have been collected and arranged in a systematic order.

Credentials evaluation: An analysis of an individual's qualifications, for example, education and licensure documents, to ensure that they are comparable to U.S. qualifications.

Department of Labor (DOL): The U.S. government department responsible for improving working conditions and promoting opportunities for profitable employment in the United States.

Department of State (DOS): The U.S. government department that sets and maintains foreign policies, runs consular offices abroad, and makes decisions about nonimmigrant and immigrant visas that are processed through U.S. consulates.

Educational comparability: Where instructional coursework under one educational system is mostly equivalent to that of another.

Internship: Where one works as a trainee gaining practical, on-the-job experience for a specified amount of time, for example, as a new nurse graduate in a hospital critical care unit.

Labor certification: Process of proving that an employer has ensured that there are no qualified U.S. workers for the position being offered to a foreign worker.

Mentor: A senior or experienced person in a company or organization who gives guidance and training to a junior colleague; a wise and trusted teacher and counselor.

Preceptor: A specialist in a profession, especially health care, who gives practical training to a student or novice in a profession.

Prevailing wage: Defined as the hourly wage, usual benefits, and overtime paid in the largest city in each county to the majority of workers.

Union: An organization of workers who have banded together to achieve common goals in key areas such as wages, hours, and working conditions.

U.S. Citizenship and Immigration Service (USCIS): The U.S. government agency that oversees lawful immigration to the United States. It establishes immigration services, policies, and priorities and **adjudicates** the petitions and applications of potential immigrants.

Since World War II, foreign-educated nurses have played a vital role in the U.S. health care system. They have augmented the workforce during periods of shortage and continue to be an essential part of the U.S. nursing profession. However, migratory patterns always have been tied to U.S. immigration policy, with changes based on environmental, economic, and political considerations. This chapter will discuss the history of foreign-educated nurses in the United States and the U.S. immigration policies that influenced that history. It will identify the challenges faced during transition to U.S. nursing practice and how they can be minimized and discuss the process of effective acculturation.

U.S. IMMIGRATION PATTERNS

Since its founding, the United States has depended on workers from other countries to provide the labor and skills necessary to ensure development of the U.S. agricultural, manufacturing, and export industries. Early immigrant workers ranged from indentured servants and African and Caribbean slaves to Irish, Italian, and Polish mill and mine workers and Chinese railroad builders. Today, the face of the immigrant is changing.

Early Immigration Trends

While immigration has been ongoing since the time of the early U.S. settlers, the United States experienced a major wave of immigration in the 1800s as people began leaving their home countries because of crop failures, land and job shortages, rising taxes, and famine. Many came to the United States because it was seen to be the land of economic opportunity. Others came seeking personal freedom or relief from political and religious persecution. The majority of immigrants during this intense period of immigration arrived from Germany, Ireland, and England.

Migration Trends in the 20th Century

Migration patterns changed considerably in the 1900s. Not only did the number of immigrants increase, but the countries from which they came also changed—with the majority of immigrants coming from non–English-speaking European countries. The principal source of immigrants was now southern and eastern Europe, especially Italy, Poland, and Russia, countries quite different in culture and language from the then-population of the United States, making adaptation to the new country more challenging than for previous immigrants.

Although each ethnic group demonstrated distinctive characteristics, they shared one overarching feature: They settled in urban areas and worked in jobs that native-born Americans were prohibited from applying for or did not want. In fact, they made up the bulk of the U.S. industrial labor pool, making possible the emergence of such industries as steel, coal, automobile, textile, and garment production and enabling the United States to move to the front ranks of the world's economic giants.

By the mid-1900s, migration patterns changed again. Restriction of immigration occurred sporadically over the course of the late 19th and early 20th centuries, but immediately after World War I (1914–1918) and into the early 1920s, Congress changed the nation's basic policy on immigration (Library of Congress, 2004).

Legislating Immigration

National Origins Act

The National Origins Act (also known as the Reed-Johnson Act) of 1924 not only restricted the number of immigrants who could enter the United States but also assigned slots according to quotas based on national origins. The Act limited the number of immigrants who could be admitted from any country to 2% of the number of persons from that country who were already living in the United States based on the 1890 census. Approximately 86% of the 165,000 permitted entries were from the British Isles, France, Germany, and other northern European countries.

The law was aimed at further restricting the southern and eastern Europeans who had begun to enter the country in large numbers beginning in the 1890s. However, it set no limits on immigration from the Western hemisphere, thus ushering in a new era in U.S. immigration history. Immigrants could and did move quite freely from Mexico, the Caribbean (including Jamaica, Barbados, and Haiti), and other parts of Central and South America.

Immigration and Nationality Act

The Immigration and Nationality Act (INA) was created in 1952. Before the INA, a variety of rulings governed immigration law but were not organized in one location. The INA collected and **codified** many existing provisions and reorganized the structure of immigration law. The Act has been amended many times over the years, but it is still the basic body of immigration law. The INA of 1952 upheld the national origins quota system established by the National Origins Act of 1924, reinforcing this controversial system of immigrant selection.

The Hart-Celler Act

Immigration policy changed with passage of the Hart-Celler Act of 1965. This Act was an amendment to the INA and was a by-product of the civil rights revolution and a much more liberal immigration law.

The Hart-Celler Act replaced the quota system with preference categories based on family relationships and job skills, giving particular preference to potential immigrants with relatives in the United States and with occupations deemed critical by the U.S. **Department of Labor (DOL).** Immigrants were to be admitted on the basis of their skills and professions rather than their nationality.

Immigration Today

The result of the Hart-Celler Act was that most legal immigrants now come to the United States from Asia and Latin America, rather than Europe. The Act also began the rejuvenation of the Asian American community in the United States by abolishing the strict quotas that had restricted immigration from Asia since 1882. After 1970, following an initial influx from European countries, immigrants began to come to the United States from countries such as Korea, China, India, the Philippines, and Pakistan, as well as countries in Africa, such as Nigeria, Egypt, and Ethiopia. By the beginning of the 21st century, immigration to the United States had returned to its previous volume in the 1900s, and the United States once again became a nation formed and transformed by immigrants.

HISTORY OF FOREIGN-EDUCATED NURSES IN THE U.S. WORKFORCE

U.S. immigration policy has evolved over time to respond to the country's need for not only various labor skills but also health care delivery. Foreign-educated nurses have been a part of the U.S. workforce since the 1940s. However, their recruitment has ebbed and waned as the health care system has been challenged by demographic and economic changes and changing immigration laws.

Legislating Nurse Immigration

Because of cyclical and often severe nursing shortages, several immigration laws and regulations were implemented to facilitate the migration of foreign-educated nurses to the United States, and many foreign-educated nurses were designated with special status. Still others were considered *persons of distinguished merit and ability*, a designation that resulted in open-ended stays in the United States but unfortunately led to an abuse of the temporary visas. In the late 1980s, it was discovered that there were upwards of 27,000 nurses who had been allowed to stay longer than 5 years even though their visas were temporary. Because of these issues, Congress not only tightened the oversight of nursing visas but also granted amnesty to some nurses because of the adverse impact the deportation of foreign-educated nurses would have on major hospitals and emergency care. The Immigration Nursing Relief Act of 1989 was the outcome of discussions among Congress, hospitals, nursing organizations, and **unions.**

Immigration Nursing Relief Act

The Immigration Nursing Relief Act of 1989 created the H-1A visa category for registered nurses for a period of 5 years. There were no limits placed on the number of nurses who could enter the United States under this visa category, a move that was intended to relieve the nursing shortage of the 1980s.

Also under the Immigration Nursing Relief Act, the DOL established a special category, referred to as *Schedule A*, in recognition of the continuing shortage of registered nurses and physical therapists. Schedule A continues to be in effect in the United States.

Schedule A alleviates some of the documentation required of a sponsoring employer by the DOL for its **labor certification** process. Just as immigration can be an expensive process for foreign-educated nurses, labor certification is a complicated, labor-intensive, and costly process for employers. Schedule A's core premise is to precertify those occupations for which there are few qualified, willing, and available U.S. workers. For Schedule A occupations, the **prevailing wage** determination request form that employers must complete goes directly to the **U.S. Citizenship and Immigration Service** (USCIS) for processing, bypassing DOL and streamlining the labor certification process. The Immigration Nursing Relief Act sunsetted (or expired) in 1995, which left foreign-educated nurses without a special visa category of their own and resulted in a return to the quota system of previous years.

Illegal Immigration Reform and Immigrant Responsibility Act

The enactment of the Illegal Immigration Reform and Immigrant Responsibility Act of 1996 (IIRIRA) on September 30, 1996, resulted in significant changes to existing U.S. immigration laws. Although IIRIRA was promoted as an illegal immigration law, its far-reaching provisions have had a serious impact on legal immigration as well.

The Act requires that select health care professionals, excluding physicians, seeking an occupational visa to enter the United States for employment purposes undergo a federal screening program. The law further requires that foreign nurses have their education, licensure, and experience evaluated to ensure their comparability to those of an entry-level U.S. nurse. The Commission on Graduates of Foreign Nursing Schools (CGFNS) was named in the law to conduct such a screening program and developed its VisaScreen program to meet the law's requirements (see chapter 3 for more on the 1996 law and its requirements).

Profile of Foreign-Educated Nurses in the U.S. Workforce

The history of foreign-educated nurses in the U.S. workforce mirrors the immigration seen in the United States from the early 1960s through the present time. Cumulative CGFNS data from 1978 to 2000 indicate that the majority of foreign-educated nurses seeking to migrate to the United States came from the Philippines (73%), followed by the United Kingdom (4%), India (3%), Nigeria (3%), and Ireland (3%). By 2008, that profile had changed. Data from CGFNS show that nurses educated in the Philippines continue to be in the majority, but the overall percentage declined from 73% to 59%—while the percentage of nurses educated in India increased from 3% to 19%. Canada (5%) and the Republic of Korea (3%) are now among the top countries of education of nurses seeking an occupational visa, while the number of nurses coming from the United Kingdom and Ireland has declined (CGFNS International, 2008).

Registered Nurses

Registered nurses entering the United States for purposes of employment tend to be female, younger than their U.S. counterparts, and educated in either diploma or baccalaureate programs in their home countries. They are generally licensed in their home countries and have worked for a number of years before migrating to the United States. First-level general nurses are known in the United States as registered nurses and are entitled to use the designation RN after their names once they pass the NCLEX-RN® examination. Foreign-educated RNs tend to work predominantly in hospitals in the areas of critical care and adult health (CGFNS, 2002).

The 2004 National Sample Survey of Registered Nurses (Bureau of Health Professions, 2004) indicated that the number of RNs who received their education outside of the United States increased by about 1.3% between 2000 and 2004. Nearly 90% (89.2%, or 89,860) of foreign-educated RNs were employed in nursing, with the majority concentrated in a handful of states in 2004. Nearly 70% of foreign-educated RNs worked in six states:

- California (28.6%)
- Florida (10.7%)
- New York (10.4%)
- Texas (7.5%)
- New Jersey (6.9%)
- Illinois (5.6%)

The survey also found that foreign-educated RNs are more likely than the U.S. RN population overall to be employed in hospitals (64.7% versus 56.2% of employed RNs overall) and more likely to be staff nurses (72.6% versus 59.1% of employed RNs overall).

Licensed Practical Nurses

Foreign-educated nurses entering the U.S. licensed practical nurse workforce tend to be female, older than their U.S. counterparts, and educated in either secondary or post-secondary nursing programs in their home countries. They maintain nursing licensure in their native lands and have practiced nursing for several years prior to immigrating to the United States. The majority of those educated as practical nurses come from Canada, Haiti, Jamaica, and Kenya.

Second-level, or enrolled nurses, are known in the United States as practical nurses. Once they achieve U.S. licensure, they receive the title licensed practical nurse or LPN. The U.S. licensure examination for practical nurses is different from that for registered nurses and is known as the NCLEX-PN® examination. To be eligible for the NCLEX-PN examination, the individual must have graduated from a government approved, practical nurse program. It should be noted, however, that many nurses who were educated as RNs in their home country have taken the NCLEX-PN examination in the United States. This has occurred for two reasons: (1) their education as a first-level general nurse was not deemed comparable to the education of an RN in the United States, or (2) the nurse was unable to pass the NCLEX-RN examination and then sat for the NCLEX-PN examination, which is allowed in some states.

The majority of those working as LPNs in the United States work in long-term care facilities, followed by hospitals and home health agencies. When working in hospitals, LPNs tend to work in gerontology and adult health. Most LPNs work in the state of New York, followed by the states of New Jersey, Florida, Texas, and Illinois (CGFNS, 2005).

Establishment of CGFNS

In the late 1960s and early 1970s, the United States was facing a critical nursing shortage. Large numbers of foreign-educated nurses were being recruited to the United States by employers and recruiting agencies. Unfortunately, only 15%–20% of those nurses were able to pass the State Board Test Pool Exam (SBTPE), the then-licensure examination for U.S. nurses. Those who failed the exam could not work as registered nurses. They either returned home to their country of origin or were employed as technicians, medical assistants, or nurse's aides. In some instances, dishonest employers expected those who were employed in such a capacity to perform the functions of an RN. However, the nurses did not have the protection of licensure and were being paid less than RN wages. These unlicensed personnel and their employers were violating states' laws—laws that prohibit the practice of nursing without a state license.

Government Review

These circumstances came to the attention of the federal government. In 1972, the Secretaries of the DOL and the Department of Health, Education, and Welfare (HEW) engaged the American Nurses Association (ANA) and Pace University to study the issue, and the findings were published in 1975. Subsequently, a conference of stakeholders was called by HEW. The participants were the DOL, the **Department of State (DOS),** the Immigration and Naturalization Service (INS), the American Hospital Association (AHA), and several nursing organizations. The participants assessed whether or not a preliminary examination could be used to predict a nurse's potential to pass the SBTPE, which was administered by the individual states with various minimum score requirements.

The idea of a predictor examination administered overseas seemed logical for two reasons: (1) foreign-educated nurses could determine if they were eligible for the U.S. licensure examination and if they had a reasonable chance of passing it before they left their home countries, and (2) potential employers could determine the nurse's potential to be U.S. licensed before he or she was sponsored for a visa.

CGFNS Origins

The conference finally recommended that a predictor exam be established and administered by a single, independent body. For this purpose, the CGFNS was created in 1977. CGFNS was initially co-funded by ANA and the National League for Nursing (NLN) as well as by a grant from the W. K. Kellogg Foundation. CGFNS was established to validate and evaluate the credentials and nursing knowledge of foreign-educated nurses in order to minimize adverse incidents, to ensure safe care to the public, and to provide a stable workforce for employers.

At that time, CGFNS was housed at the Educational Commission on Foreign Medical Graduates (ECFMG) in Philadelphia, Pennsylvania. ECFMG had been performing a similar screening function for foreign-educated medical graduates who wanted to practice as physicians in the United States. CGFNS adopted the concepts of **credentials evaluation** and **educational comparability** used by ECFMG.

CGFNS Today

CGFNS is an immigration-neutral, nonprofit organization, internationally recognized as an authority on credentials evaluation related to the education, registration, and licensure of nurses and other health care professionals worldwide. It protects the public by ensuring that nurses and other health care professionals educated in countries other than the United States are eligible and qualified to meet licensure, immigration, and other practice requirements in the United States. CGFNS not only validates international professional credentials but also supports international regulatory and educational standards for health care professionals.

CGFNS Programs

CGFNS has four programs that are used by foreign-educated nurses to meet federal and state requirements for employment as a nurse in the United States: the VisaScreen program, the Certification Program, the Credentials Evaluation Service, and the New York Credentials Verification Service. The VisaScreen program is required for nurses seeking an occupational visa to work as a nurse in the United States. The visa gives entry into the country. To work as a nurse, you must have a license to practice in a particular state. The license is granted by the State Board of Nursing in the intended state of practice. Many State Boards of Nursing require foreign-educated nurses to have their nursing credentials (education and licensure) reviewed, their nursing knowledge evaluated, and their English language proficiency scores verified by CGFNS as a prerequisite for state licensure (see chapter 4). The individual State Board of Nursing will advise you as to their CGFNS requirements. Generally, states use one of the four CGFNS programs:

- *Certification Program* (CP), which includes a review of your secondary school and nursing education; verification of your initial licensure in your country of education as well as your current licensure; the CGFNS Qualifying Exam; and an English-language proficiency examination;
- *Credentials Evaluation Service* (CES), which provides a written analysis of your education and licensure in terms of U.S. comparability;
- *VisaScreen program,* which is a government-mandated program ensuring that your education, licensure, and experience are comparable to those of U.S. graduates; that your license is valid, current, and without penalties; that you have proficiency in written and oral English; and that, if you are a registered

nurse, you have passed a test of nursing knowledge, either the CGFNS Qualifying Exam or the NCLEX-RN examination; or

■ *New York Credentials Verification Service* (NYCVS), which obtains your academic transcripts and licensure validations from the issuing agencies, verifies their authenticity, and provides a report to the New York State Department of Education. The state then evaluates your credentials to determine comparability to U.S. education and licensure.

State Licensure

Unlike countries that have a national licensure system, licensure in the United States is at the state level, and each state sets its own requirements. You cannot work in the United States without a nursing license, therefore, you should contact the Board of Nursing in your intended state of practice as soon as possible to determine the requirements for that state before you begin the licensure process (see chapter 4 for more information on state licensure). Success on the U.S. licensure examination is linked to the amount of time that has passed since you graduated from nursing school. The shorter the time between graduation from your school of nursing and taking the NCLEX-RN examination, the greater the chance of passing the exam (CGFNS, 2007). Once you are licensed in your state of intended practice and ready for employment, there are many ways in which you can move smoothly to nursing practice in the United States.

TRANSITION TO NURSING PRACTICE IN THE UNITED STATES

Beginning nursing practice in a new country can be both exciting and challenging. You will meet new colleagues and friends, and you will be introduced to a new health care system and new technologies. Initially, you may feel intimidated, but over time you will begin to understand the new system and how nursing care is provided within that system.

Navigating immigration, moving to the United States, obtaining state licensure, and becoming comfortable in a health care system different from your own can be a lengthy, sometimes challenging process—a process that balances the needs of migrating nurses with protection of the U.S. public. However, meeting the challenges of migration provides unlimited career opportunities.

Orientation to Practice

Preparation is critical to safe practice, therefore, hospitals and other employing facilities want the foreign-educated nurse to succeed and are willing to create an orientation that truly facilitates each nurse's transition to U.S. practice. It is your responsibility to let orientation leaders know how effective the orientation is, answering such questions as: What made sense and what did not? Did you need more information about or assistance with a specific aspect of nursing care? Did you need more time to process the information? In other words, do not be afraid to speak up so that the orientation is meaningful for you.

Support Systems

Another factor that is crucial to having a smooth transition to practice is having a support system in place. Support systems have been identified by nurse executives as vital to an international nurse's ability to adapt to nursing practice in the United States (Davis, 2004). Be sure to ask if the hospital has an **internship** program for international nurses, or if the hospital will provide you with a **preceptor** to assist you through the transition period. The delivery of nursing care in the United States can be complex and challenging. For many foreign-educated nurses it is the first time to manage a group of patients and use unfamiliar technology. A **mentor** or preceptor can guide you through the transition and help you to understand how hospital processes relate to each other, thus ensuring safe practice. A mentor is a senior or experienced person in a company or organization who gives guidance and training to a junior colleague. A mentor is considered a wise and trusted teacher and counselor. The mentor relationship is not limited to a specific task or timeframe but generally lasts over a period of years. A preceptor is a specialist in a profession, especially health care, who gives practical training to a student or novice in a profession. The relationship may or may not last after completion of the period of preceptorship.

Challenges During Transition

Most foreign-educated nurses work in hospital settings when they first come to the United States, typically specializing in adult health and critical care; therefore, an awareness of the challenges of entering nursing practice in the United States can be helpful. While most nurses look forward to working in the United States, adjustment to practice can be affected by several factors, such as the health care system of the nurse's home country, language competence, knowledge of medications and their administration, and familiarity with technology (Edwards & Davis, 2006).

Variations in Health Care Systems

The more similar your health care system is to that of the United States, the easier your transition and the more comfortable you will be in the clinical setting. You can then focus on specific practice needs rather than the transition process. Information about the U.S. health care system is cited most frequently as a necessary component of clinical orientation by foreign-educated nurses. Because health care systems vary greatly from country to country, it is essential that you have an understanding of how the U.S. system works. This includes a description of the health team, its members, and their roles. Information on health insurance and how the system is accessed by patients also should be included. Although you will not come to understand the system thoroughly until you work within it, preliminary knowledge helps to make the transition to U.S. practice less stressful.

Language Competency

Nurses for whom English is a second language have repeatedly indicated to CGFNS that perception of their nursing competence by patients and health care personnel is tied to their ability to speak

English. Employers cite language competence as the most critical skill that foreign-educated nurses need during their first year of practice in the United States.

If English is a second language for you, it is best to increase your English language skills as you transition to living and practicing in the United States. Language skills, like practice skills, are primarily obtained through experience. Exercise your language skills by using English as much as possible in your new environment, even if it makes you feel uncomfortable or embarrassed at first. If you do not understand a term, ask for clarification. Look for publications that describe the idioms, abbreviations, and slang terms used in nursing practice in the United States.

Most of all, do not feel that you have to apologize to your employer or your colleagues for your attempts at using this new language. If you ask for help, most staff will try to help you to understand the nuances of the language. If one colleague does not take the time to assist you, it does not mean that others will react in the same way. While it may be difficult to say, "I don't understand what you mean," it is the only way to begin understanding the use of words within the context of U.S. nursing care.

Knowledge of Medications and Pharmacology

Western medicine relies heavily on drugs to treat patient illness, many of which are not used in other countries. Some drugs that are available internationally have different trade names, while others may be experimental and not yet known internationally, making it difficult for the nurse entering U.S. nursing practice. Pharmacology can be intimidating, mainly because of the volume of medications given on a daily basis in the United States and the various medication routes. Most of the errors made by foreign-educated nurses in their first year of practice are related to medication administration.

Proficiency in Technology

The U.S. health care system relies heavily on technology for diagnostic, preventive, and palliative care—much more so than other countries around the world. Because foreign-educated nurses tend to work in adult health and critical care units in hospitals, they are confronted with technology on a daily basis as they transition to U.S. practice. However, international nurses participating in a joint CGFNS/ Excelsior College study on their perception of readiness for practice in the United States indicated that technology is one of the areas in which they felt least prepared (Edwards & Davis, 2006).

ACCULTURATION

Acculturation—the process of adapting or learning to take on the behaviors and attitudes of another group or culture—is an essential aspect of working in a host country. For nurses transitioning to practice in the United States, it generally takes 4 to 6 months to become fully productive and 12 months to feel fully acclimated to the new setting.

Phases of Acculturation

Acculturation can be divided into four phases: acquaintance, indignation, conflict resolution, and integration. Familiarity with the process of acculturation will help you to know what to expect within your first year of practice in a new culture and new work environment.

The *acquaintance* phase of acculturation occurs from entry into the culture to 3 months post arrival. It is the stage of initial contact, during which time you will be excited about your new life and your new place of employment. This is the time in which you will become oriented not just to the practice environment but also to the community—the time during which you will begin to develop a supportive social network of both colleagues and friends.

The *indignation* phase occurs 3 to 6 months post arrival. The feelings of excitement about your new environment give way to feelings of anxiety, which can lead to a sense of isolation and psychological discomfort. Understanding the U.S. health care system and your role in it—what is expected of you and how quickly it is expected— can become overwhelming. It is during this time that a mentor or preceptor will be critical. The support that mentors or preceptors can provide is invaluable because they have knowledge of the system and contacts within and outside of the system; most importantly, they are willing to work with you so that your experience is a positive one. This also is the time to rely on family, friends, and colleagues for support—and especially those who have been through a similar experience.

It also may be helpful to seek out regional support groups. There are support groups within the United States designed to help immigrants adapt to their new life. These support groups are generally composed of individuals of the same ethnic background who have been through the immigration and transition processes and are willing to share their experiences with those who are new to this country. The Chamber of Commerce in the city or town in which you intend to practice can provide you with a list of support services that are available.

The *conflict resolution* phase generally occurs 6 to 9 months post arrival. This is the time to clarify new roles and development, to gain insight into problem solving, and to make personal and professional decisions about your new workplace and your new community. You may feel that you are a part of two cultures—your native culture and its work values and the culture of the U.S. health care system and U.S. nursing.

Now is the time to determine what values and beliefs are essential to you. What values and knowledge from your own culture make you comfortable as a nurse in the United States? Which of the values of the new culture and the new workplace can you incorporate into your practice as a nurse? What aspects of nursing practice in the United States do you find difficult to adopt—and why? Again, exploring these issues with a mentor, a preceptor, or someone familiar with the process of adapting to a new culture and work environment will be invaluable.

The *integration* phase occurs 9 to 12 months post arrival. It is the phase of renewed enthusiasm for your work and your new country, a time when you have reconciled the differences between your native culture and your host culture, and a time when you feel confident in your ability to practice as a nurse in the new culture. It is a time when you know you made the right decision to migrate and a time when you will have a sense of belonging to the new culture and, most importantly, a sense of the skills and knowledge that you bring to the profession (Adeniran, Davis, & Nichols, 2005).

SUMMARY

The demand for nurses in the next decade is expected to increase substantially in the United States. International nurses will continue to have a significant impact on the U.S. nursing workforce and contribute to its growth. The migration of nurses across international borders and their assimilation into the U.S. workforce enables nursing to grow, to broaden its perspective, and to increase its diversity; therefore, the successful adaptation of foreign-educated nurses to U.S. practice is critical.

REFERENCES

Adeniran, R. K., Davis, C. R., & Nichols, B. L. (2005). *Empowering internationally educated nurses through collaboration.* Paper presented at the 23rd Quadrennial Congress of the International Council of Nurses, Taipei, Taiwan.

Bureau of Health Professions. (2004). *The registered nurse population: Findings from the 2004 national sample survey of registered nurses.* Retrieved February 12, 2009, from http://bhpr.hrsa.gov/healthworkforce/rnsurvey04/.

CGFNS International. (2008). VisaScreen statistical data. Retrieved February 12, 2009, from http://www.cgfns.org/sections/tools/stats/vs.shtml.

The Commission on Graduates of Foreign Nursing Schools. (2002). *Characteristics of foreign nurse graduates in the United States workforce.* Philadelphia: Author.

The Commission on Graduates of Foreign Nursing Schools. (2005). *Characteristics of international practical nurses in the United States workforce.* Philadelphia: Author.

The Commission on Graduates of Foreign Nursing Schools. (2007). CGFNS validity study 2006–2007. Unpublished statistical report.

Davis, C. R. (2004, February/March). Crossing borders: International nurses in the U.S. workforce. *Imprint, 51*(2), 49–51.

Edwards, P., & Davis, C. (2006, November/December). International nurses perceptions of their clinical practice. *Journal of Continuing Education in Nursing, 37*(6), 265–269.

Library of Congress. (2004). *American memory timeline: Rise of industrial America, 1876–1900.* Retrieved February 9, 2009, from http://memory.loc.gov/learn/features/timeline/riseind/immgnts/immgrnts.html

2

Preparing to Leave Your Home Country

CATHERINE R. DAVIS
DONNA R. RICHARDSON

In This Chapter

Nurse Migration Factors

Before You Leave Your Home Country

Choosing a Recruiter

Remittances

Summary

Resources

Keywords

Acculturation program: A system of procedures or activities that has the specific purpose of training individuals to understand another culture and its practices.

Advocacy: Active support for a cause or position.

Breach of contract: A legal concept in which a binding agreement is *not* honored by one or more of the participants.

Codes of Conduct: Sets of rules outlining the responsibilities of, or proper practices for, individuals or the members of an organization or profession.

Continuing education: Regular courses or training designed to bring professionals up to date with the latest developments in their particular field.

Department of Homeland Security (DHS): A U.S. government agency created in 2003 to handle immigration and other security-related matters. A component of DHS is the Citizenship and Immigration Services, the government agency that oversees lawful immigration to the United States.

Garnished wages: Monies taken from payroll or royalty checks, or from investment checks, to pay a debt.

Pen pals: Two people, usually in different countries, who become friends through an exchange of letters but who may never meet.

Portfolio: A collection of items or documents outlining one's work experience, achievements, and skills organized in a binder, file, or electronic format.

Remittances: The portion of migrant income that, in the form of either funds or goods, goes back into the home country.

Residency programs: Positions wherein one works for a specific period of time in a community or a facility to gain experience. In many U.S. facilities such programs are structured learning experiences.

Self-learning modules: Activities designed for participants to undertake independently when they are unable to attend traditional education sessions.

Migration is the movement of people across borders, usually for the purpose of acquiring a new residence and employment. Migration can occur within countries (internal) or across national borders (external). The annual flow of international migration has continued to increase over the past decades so that in the early 21st century it is estimated that 1 out of every 35 individuals worldwide is an inter-national migrant (Kingma, 2006).

NURSE MIGRATION FACTORS

People have many reasons for migrating—usually identified as push factors (reasons for leaving their own country) and pull factors (reasons for choosing a host country). Push factors may include such things as poor wages, poor working conditions, civil war, or other factors that make living and working in a country difficult. Pull factors are those that make a host country desirable and include such things as higher wages, greater professional opportunities, and better work environments.

Push/Pull Factors

The world is seeing a sharp increase in the number of highly skilled workers moving across international borders (Kingma, 2006). Health care professionals, including nurses, make up a significant portion of that increase. In a CGFNS survey (2007), foreign-educated nurses in the United States most frequently cited poor wages and few jobs as the primary reasons for leaving their home countries (push factors). The United States was identified as the destination of choice because of such pull factors as better wages and working conditions, a better way of life, and greater opportunity for advancement. Many nurses responding to the survey had family members living in the United States, and this also was cited as a pull factor.

Since the mid-1900s, nurses educated outside the United States have augmented the U.S. workforce during periods of shortage. Today, nursing is one of the fastest growing U.S. professions, but the United States is experiencing a nursing shortage that is expected to reach as much as 800,000 by the year 2020 (Pittman, Folsom, Bass, & Leonhardy, 2007). However, migration patterns and the availability of international nurses often change based on environmental, economic, and political considerations. As a result of the aging of its general population and an aging nurse workforce, the United States is facing a major nursing shortage.

Projections for the Future

The U.S. Department of Health and Human Services (HHS) estimates that there will be a shortage of 800,000 registered nurses by 2020 (Department of Health and Human Services, 2002). It is against this backdrop that the recruitment of foreign-educated nurses must be viewed. During the past 50 years, the United States has regularly recruited foreign-educated nurses for employment in a wide variety of settings. What differs today is the rise of global, profit-seeking recruitment agencies specializing in international recruitment and an increasing number of countries educating nurses for export (Brush, Sochalski, & Berger, 2004). The continued nursing shortage in the United States and the proliferation of foreign nurse recruitment agencies suggest that foreign-educated nurses will continue to be a viable part of the U.S. nurse workforce.

BEFORE YOU LEAVE YOUR HOME COUNTRY

Leaving one's home county is a significant event—one that produces many changes in your life. Leaving your home, family, and friends to move to a new land can be daunting, but understanding the migration process, knowing what to expect, and being aware of your rights can smooth the transition and make it a worthwhile experience.

Becoming a nurse in the United States begins with seeking an occupational visa, which will allow you entry into the country for the purpose of employment. Canadian and Mexican nurses may obtain trade NAFTA (North American Free Trade Agreement) status for this purpose. A description of the different types of visas available to nurses seeking to come to the United States is outlined in chapter 3 of this publication.

Embracing Life in a New Culture

When you decide to immigrate to the United States, the initial excitement of the decision can fade into a stressful, worrisome time when you realize you have to not only embrace a new life and culture but also say goodbye to family and friends. One of the most important tasks when deciding to move abroad is to get your family and friends involved in the decisions you are making. Often close family feel left out and worried that they do not know what choices you are making. Involving family and friends by discussing with them possible places to live, areas to visit in the United States, and other aspects of your new life can help to allay their concerns. It allows them to see that you are putting plenty of thought into your actions and that their opinions are important to you.

Often the biggest decision when emigrating is the initial one, when you decide where you would like to work and when you would like to move. While immigration procedures may affect the timing of your move to the United States, there still are numerous steps you will need to go through in order to have a successful and relatively stress-free move. The best way of ensuring that you have taken care of everything is to prepare a "To Do" list. That way you can take the time to organize the move, identify what needs to be done, check off the completed items, and know what still needs to be accomplished. If nothing else, this should give you a sense of control over the process. Following are some of the steps you will have to take when considering moving to the United States.

Choosing Where You Want to Live

The United States is composed of many geographic regions, each with its own climate, culture, and customs. For example, the Middle Atlantic states of Pennsylvania, New York, and New Jersey enjoy four distinct seasons of the year (summer, fall, winter, and spring). These states were among the original 13 British colonies that became the United States and are rich in historical tradition. They each include densely populated, major cities with large, ethnically diverse communities and many rural towns and communities. By contrast, California, a Pacific state, contains areas that are considered ideal resort destinations, sunny and dry all year with easy access to the ocean and mountains. California's historical and cultural traditions reflect its origins as part of Mexico prior to gaining U.S. statehood in 1850.

Determining where you want to live is a major decision that may be influenced by the choices of nurses who have migrated before you. CGFNS (2002) examined the characteristics of foreign-educated nurses in the U.S. workforce and found that New York, California, Texas, Florida, and Illinois were the major states of nurse immigration. Canadian nurses most often resided in Texas, followed by Florida, North Carolina, California, and Michigan. Filipino nurses resided primarily in California, followed by Illinois, Hawaii, New Jersey, and New York. Nurses educated in India were located primarily in California, Illinois, New York, and Texas.

Questions to Ask

Because of the wide geographic diversity in the United States, you should use a library or the Internet to research the different areas of the country and ask yourself such questions as:

- Do I want to live in a climate that is similar to my home country or experience something different?
- Do I want to live in a large city, small city, town, or rural community?
- Do I want to live where I already have friends and family, or do I want to be on my own?
- Do I want to live in a mountainous area, a plains area, or by the ocean?
- Do I want to live close to my employing institution? How do I want to commute? By auto? By public transportation?
- How will I make living arrangements? Who will meet me when I arrive? How will I get to my destination?

Choosing the Type of Employment Facility

Prior to leaving your home country, you should consider the type of U.S. facility in which you would like to work. Foreign-educated nurses in all regions of the United States most frequently are employed in hospitals, followed by smaller percentages in long-term care facilities (such as nursing homes), ambulatory care settings, community health, and home health. Those employed in hospital settings work primarily in adult health and critical care.

Questions to Ask

Questions you might consider prior to employment are:

- Do I want to work in a hospital or another type of facility?
- Do I want to work in the community as opposed to a structured facility?
- Do I want to work in a rural or urban area?
- Do I want to work in a small hospital (100 beds) or a large facility (300+ beds)?
- Do I want to work in a public (government-operated) facility, such as a Veterans Administration Hospital, or in a private (nongovernment) facility?
- Do I want to work in a teaching or nonteaching facility? Teaching hospitals serve as training sites for new physicians during their internship and **residency programs.** These hospitals are usually affiliated with a medical school and may be part of an academic health center that includes other health professional schools, including nursing schools.
- What specialty areas do I enjoy most (adult health, critical care, maternal infant, pediatrics, etc.)?
- In what areas of nursing am I most skilled or proficient?

Selecting a Health Care Facility

Once you have identified potential places of employment, you should carefully research their hiring practices, the units and shifts available, the orientation provided, and the placement of foreign-educated nurses.

Questions to Ask

Questions to consider prior to accepting a nursing position are:

- Do I have to sign a **contract?** What is the length of the contract? What does the contract require me to do? What is the penalty if I break the contract?

- To what unit will I be assigned? Will I have to move from unit to unit, as needed? How large is the unit? How many patients will I be responsible for at a time?
- To what shift will I be assigned (day, evening, night), and what will be the length of the shift (8 hours, 10 hours, or 12 hours)? How much overtime will I be expected to work? Is overtime mandatory?
- What will my salary be? Is my salary comparable to what other nurses are earning?
- Will my nursing experience in my home country be considered in my starting salary, my starting position, and in promotion? How often will my performance be evaluated?
- What type of orientation will be provided? How will it be modified to meet my needs? Will I be assigned a mentor or preceptor and for how long?
- Is there a "**pen pal**" or "buddy system" in place that I can access prior to leaving my home country? Is there a nurse working in the facility with whom I can correspond?

Some of these questions may be addressed by doing an Internet search, while others will have to be asked during the interview process with the specific facility.

Mentors and Preceptors

CGFNS (2005) found that employers considered preceptorship as having the greatest impact on a successful transition to U.S. practice. Employers also indicated that, on average, it took foreign-educated nurses 4 to 6 months to feel comfortable with nursing in the United States and to exhibit safe nursing practice. For those reasons alone, you should ask if a preceptor will be available to you and for how long.

A preceptor can help you understand the U.S. health care system, to become acquainted with other staff, to understand the technology used in practice, and to understand the medication administration system. A preceptor also can support you when you give your patient report to the next shift, show you how to best organize your care, and explain how to get the supplies you need. Most of all, a preceptor can help you to problem solve and can be there when you need some support.

Mastering English

The second most critical factor identified by employers as essential for foreign-educated nurses during their first year of practice was good English language skills. If English is your second language, try to improve your skills prior to leaving your home country, either through classes or **self-learning modules.** When deciding on your U.S. place of employment, ask if the facility offers any English language classes during orientation. A preceptor also may be able to assist you with your language skills, especially with the language of nursing practice in the United States (see chapter 8 on communication).

Researching the Environment

Knowing what to expect ahead of time can be critical to your adjustment in the U.S. work setting. Do not hesitate to ask the facility for a brochure or even a video of the facility, the unit on which you will work, and the staff with whom you will work. Send pictures or a video of yourself (after you have been offered and accepted employment) so the staff will be familiar with you when you arrive.

Ask for a description of the types and severity of patient conditions that you will encounter as well as the commonly represented cultures of patients and staff members.

Ask if the facility would be interested in information on your culture. The more information you and the unit staff share ahead of time, the more comfortable you will feel when beginning your nursing career in the United States.

Preparing for U.S. Licensure

To enter the United States for the purpose of employment, you will need an occupational visa, which allows you entry into the country. However, in order to practice nursing in the United States, you must have a license in the state in which you plan to work. Each state sets its own requirements for licensure, so it is important to understand those requirements and to start the process early (see chapter 4 for information on entering the U.S. workforce).

Developing Your Portfolio

A **portfolio** is a collection of items or documents outlining work experience, achievements, and skills. It is organized in a binder, file, or electronic format. By collecting and storing this information throughout your nursing career, you will become more aware of the skills and abilities you possess, and have an excellent way to market your qualifications to an employer.

A portfolio does two major things: (1) creating it helps you to focus on the milestones of your career, allows you to look back and review your accomplishments, helps you to set goals for your future, and helps to identify what will be needed to achieve those goals; and (2) presenting your portfolio to prospective employers tells the employer that you are serious about your nursing career and its advancement, that you are reflective and organized, and that you have identified a career path. The portfolio allows employers to identify your competencies, to design an orientation program that best meets your needs, and to work with you to achieve your identified goals.

A portfolio can be in hard copy, electronic, or both. Electronic portfolios can be designed as Web pages and posted to an Internet location or stored on a CD-ROM, computer wand (flash drive), or DVD, to be used as a tool to supplement the hard-copy version of your portfolio. Documents stored electronically should be printed out as needed for employment, academic admission, licensure, and other purposes. Portfolio development consists of a number of steps:

Step 1. Consider your career thus far and determine what you consider to be the most important and most significant achievements of your career so far.

Step 2. Collect all representative documents that showcase your academic and professional accomplishments and organize them into sections: for example, education, work experience, publications and presentations, memberships, **continuing education,** and awards. You might also provide a separate section for your short-term and long-term goals. Documents can be organized chronologically, from the beginning of your career to the present time.

Step 3. Create a paper file by making copies of original documents. Retain the originals and provide the copies when presenting your portfolio. If you choose to create an electronic portfolio, scan the documents onto a CD-ROM, DVD, or flash drive. Back-up files should be created on your personal computer. Copies of documents collected for portfolios include, but are not limited to:

- Academic experiences, for example, transcripts, special reports you developed, presentations you gave, copies of positive faculty evaluations, skills assessments, and summaries of research projects you completed;
- Work-related documents, such as letters of recommendation, performance evaluations, special recognitions, and copies of employee newsletters in which you are mentioned;
- Community activities that you conducted or in which you participated;
- Awards you received, for example, scholarships, academic citations, and newspaper articles noting special honors or activities;
- Letters of recommendation;
- A list of your short-term and long-term goals; and
- An updated résumé and cover letter (see Appendix A).

Step 4. Review your completed portfolio to make sure that it is accurate and concise and contains only necessary items. Make sure that it is easy to follow and tells a positive story about you. A portfolio should contain no more than 15–20 pages.

CHOOSING A RECRUITER

Approximately half of the nurses seeking to enter the United States for employment purposes use a recruiter to assist them through the migration process—from obtaining a U.S. work visa to attaining employment in a U.S. facility. The recruiter can be hospital-based (usually a nurse with experience in recruitment who is an employee of the hospital) or commercial. Commercial recruiters generally charge a fee for their services and work independently or as part of a recruitment firm. Health care recruiters report that 90% of their revenue comes from registered nurse recruitment, 3% from licensed practical nurse recruitment, and negligible amounts from the recruitment of other health professionals (Pittman et al., 2007). If you plan on using a recruiter, you should choose that recruiter carefully because the nurse recruitment industry is largely unregulated.

What to Look for in a Recruiter

Because of the global nursing shortage there has been a proliferation of commercial recruiters here in the United States and worldwide. There are many recruiters whose policies are transparent (visible and clear) and who use best practices. They often also provide transition and **acculturation programs** to ensure the acceptance and comfort of their nurses in their new employment positions. Several recruitment companies have participated in the development of **Codes of Conduct** for recruiters and employers through collaboration with policymakers, unions, nursing organizations, and employers (Pittman et al., 2007).

On the other hand, there are some recruiting firms that are poorly funded and often require foreign-educated nurses to pay for their own examination review courses and travel expenses. Reportedly, some recruiters have solicited duplicate fees—demanding payment from nurses in addition to charging employers fees for each recruited nurse. Some recruiters, including health care recruiters, have made unfulfilled promises, misrepresented positions and resources, or charged unwarranted fees, therefore, you should investigate your recruiter carefully before agreeing to be their client.

Finding a Recruiter

Currently, there is not a public site for reviewing the ethical conduct of recruitment companies, but there are efforts underway for the development of a user-based review system whereby clients can make public comments regarding their experience with nurse recruiters. Until such a service is available, you should contact friends and colleagues to determine what recruiters they used and if their experiences with the recruiter were positive. Check Internet postings about the recruiter you are considering, and check to see if the recruiter is a member of the National Association of Healthcare Recruiters (NAHCR) or the American Association of International Healthcare Recruitment.

Rights and Responsibilities of Nurse Recruits

Nurses using a recruiting firm to assist with the process of migration have the right to be treated fairly and equitably, to review their contract before signing, to not have their contract modified unless agreed upon by both parties, and to have their interaction with recruiters free from intimidation. Recruiting firms commonly are founded by immigrants themselves, or by individuals who previously lived overseas and are familiar with the language and business opportunities in the source countries (Pittman et al., 2007). Although you may feel more comfortable with a recruiter of the same ethnic background as yours, you should still carefully investigate that recruiter's reputation—just as you would with any recruiter—prior to signing a contract. Ask for the recruiter's references, that is, names of recruited nurses and of health care institutions that have hired nurses recruited by that firm. Do not rely on spoken promises. Request written documentation of all details.

Knowing Your Rights

Nurses have the responsibility of knowing their rights before they leave their home country and of finding out as much as possible about the immigration process of the host country, in this case the United States. Visit the Web site for the U.S. Department of State, which issues visas (www.state.gov). Visit the U.S. Embassy in your country or view its Internet site (which can be located through www.usembassy.gov) to gather information on the United States and its visas. Use the **Department of Homeland Security** (www.dhs.gov) and the U.S.

Citizenship and Immigration Service (USCIS; www.uscis.gov) Web sites to gain an understanding of the requirements for immigration.

Signing Contracts

The majority of recruiters have foreign-educated nurses sign contracts prior to beginning the immigration process. You must understand that if you sign a contract, you may be legally required to abide by all the terms of the contract. Those contracts may be legally enforceable and can mean significant monetary penalties and even deportation if violated or broken. Therefore, you should read everything carefully before signing, and you should not sign anything without taking sufficient time to review it. If you do not understand the terms of the contract, ask to have them explained until you thoroughly understand what you are signing. It may be best to have an outside attorney (an attorney not employed by the recruiter) or a trusted family member or friend read the contract before you sign it. Do not sign a contract that you cannot explain to others or that you do not understand.

Reviewing Your Contract

You have the right to receive a copy of the contract prior to signing so that you can review it. You also have the right to a signed copy of the contract for your records. Contracts should:

- Be in writing and should describe the roles and responsibilities of the recruiter as well as those of the recruited nurse;
- Outline which fees are to be paid by the recruiter and which, if any, are to be paid by the nurse;
- Identify the nurse's proposed geographic work location, place of employment, and housing, if provided; and
- Identify the length of the contract and fees charged, if any, for **breach of contract.**

Recruitment Costs

The financial costs of immigration can be high. The typical fees include visa filing fees for the visa applicant(s); medical examination fees; CGFNS program application fees; English proficiency examination fees; NCLEX examination fees; travel fees; and application costs for the state board of nursing application (varies by state). Unless your recruiter or the employer who is sponsoring your visa agrees to cover those costs and travel expenses, you will be required to pay for them directly or have them deducted from your future salary. It is important to receive a detailed account of all charges for which you will be responsible.

Breach of Contract

Generally, recruitment contracts involve a 2- to 3-year commitment and identify a "buy out" or "breach" fee that can range from $8,000 to $50,000 if the nurse recruit does not fulfill the contract. Breach fees are usually proportionate to the investment made by the recruiter in bringing the nurse to the United States and for facilitating visa, immigration, licensure, and placement processes (Pittman et al., 2007). Before signing a contract make sure that the breach fee, if any, is reasonable and will be pro-rated for the amount of work you have provided. Also ensure that if you breach your contract, you will not be required to pay the fee in one lump sum, but rather in installments. In focus groups conducted jointly by CGFNS and AcademyHealth in 2007, one Filipino nurse reported,

> I talked to my agent last Friday (who is Filipino) because I wanted to buy out my contract. My agent told me that buying out my contract would ruin his relationship with the mother company, which is one of his biggest clients. He also told me that my buying out my contract might result in revocation of my immigrant visa since it was [that company] who petitioned it. Also, if I opted to buy out, I will need to pay the whole amount in a one-time payment only, which is $13,650. For now, I can only pay them one-fourth of the buy-out price (CGFNS & AcademyHealth, 2007).

Be aware of fees for which you may have to reimburse your recruiter both during the contract and for early termination. Find out if your wages will be **garnished** (held by your employing facility and given directly to the recruiter) to reimburse the recruiter for unpaid fees, how much will be deducted from each paycheck (will your entire pay be garnished until the fees are paid, or will there be a certain percentage taken out of each paycheck?), and for what length of time the garnishment will extend.

Pitfalls and How to Avoid Them

Nurse immigrants commonly report several types of contract violations by some recruiters and employing institutions. These violations typically include: forced changes in the place or location of employment; changes from being direct hires of the facility (which is preferred by most foreign-educated nurses) to employees of staffing agencies; lower salaries than anticipated, or being paid less than U.S. nurses, which is illegal; and restricted or lacking benefits, including health insurance, vacation time, or sick leave (Pittman et al., 2007). Immigrant nurses have reported being threatened with deportation for not adhering to contracts—as well as having their VisaScreen certificates and green cards withheld by recruiters.

Recognizing Unethical Recruitment Practices

Because the nursing shortage is of such global proportion, a nurse's refusal to sign on with one recruiter will not end his or her chances to immigrate. The more information you have, the less chance that you will be intimidated or taken advantage of by recruiters or those who profess to be "immigration agents" or facilitators. Self-described "immigration agents" will falsely claim to be able to make immigration move faster for the right amount of money.

Nurses who plan to migrate to the United States can go to the U.S. Department of Labor (DOL) Web site (www.dol.gov) to access information about employment, rights of women, unions, wages, and civil rights. The DOL fosters and promotes the welfare of job seekers, wage earners, and retirees of the United States by improving their working conditions, advancing their opportunities for profitable employment, protecting their retirement and health care benefits, helping employers find workers, strengthening free collective bargaining, and tracking changes in employment, prices, and other national economic measurements. In carrying out this mission, the DOL administers a variety of Federal labor laws, including those that guarantee workers' rights to safe and healthful working conditions, a minimum hourly wage and overtime pay, freedom from employment discrimination, unemployment insurance, and other income support. There also are immigration **advocacy** groups that can provide you with reliable and correct information on U.S. immigration laws and referrals to immigration law firms.

Third-Party Authorizations

Another pitfall to be aware of is the use of third-party authorizations. These authorizations can give someone else the right to receive and open your correspondence—the right to receive your test scores, your CGFNS VisaScreen certificate, and even your green card— rather than the correspondence and documents going directly to you. Read everything carefully before signing any documents to ensure that you are not giving up rights that should be retained by you. In most cases, your signature on such a document makes it legally binding. If you believe that you have been wronged during the immigration process, seek an independent immigration attorney or civil rights attorney who can review your case with you, determine if your rights have been violated, and assist you in seeking recourse.

Ethical Recruitment of Nurses

The globalization of the nursing workforce has enabled nurses to further their careers through migration. With the increase in global migration, there has been a corresponding increase in the number of international recruiters and recruiting firms, some of whom have aggressively pursued nurses to work in developed countries. This aggressive recruitment has led, in some instances, to the serious depletion of the nurse workforce, particularly in developing countries and countries that could ill afford to lose their nurses.

In 2001, the International Council of Nurses (ICN) issued a Position Statement (revised in 2007) on ethical nurse recruitment. The Statement recognized that quality health care is directly dependent on an adequate supply of nurses in the country; it also recognized the right of the individual nurse to migrate. Most importantly, the ICN Position Statement condemned the unethical recruitment practices that have depleted nursing resources and have exploited migrating nurses. The ICN Position Statement may be found in Appendix C and accessed at http://www.icn.ch/psrecruit01.htm.

Voluntary Code of Ethical Conduct

In September 2008, a task force representing unions, health care organizations, educational and licensure bodies, and recruiters released the *Voluntary Code of Ethical Conduct for the Recruitment of Foreign-Educated Nurses to the United States* (AcademyHealth, 2008). The code aims to ensure that the growing practice of recruiting foreign-educated nurses to the United States is done in a responsible and transparent manner. The Code was developed in response to concerns that the rapid increase in international recruiting created opportunities for unethical behavior on both sides.

The Code of Conduct aims to increase transparency and accountability in international recruitment and ensure adequate orientation programs for foreign-educated nurses. It also provides guidance on ways to ensure recruitment is not harmful to the nurses' home countries. The Code is wholly voluntary. Health care organizations and recruiters that subscribe are committing to adhere to a series of practical standards and to emulate best practices (CGFNS, 2008).

REMITTANCES

One of the lessons learned from nurse migration is that nurses' source countries need to benefit as well. Foreign-educated nurses traditionally have sent **remittances** back to their home countries. Remittance refers to the portion of migrant income that, in the form of either funds or goods, goes back into the home country, primarily to support families back home, to cut poverty, and to improve education and health within the family (Focus Migration, 2006). Until 5 years ago, this transfer of funds was thought to be minor. However, nurse remittances alone increased from less than $2 billion in 1970 to over $70 billion in 1995 (Seago, 2008).

If you plan on sending money back to your family or friends, you should discuss this before you depart from your home country so that you know the best way to send money and goods. Look into fees for the transfer of money (what it will cost you to send money and what it will cost the recipient in your home country to receive it). Fees that money-sending services such as Western Union charge are usually higher than bank fees. You also should consider the security of the transfer of funds, especially if the funds are sent through more informal channels. It might be helpful to talk to someone who has migrated from your home country to the United States and is sending remittances back home. This will give you a good idea of the cost and the processes involved.

SUMMARY

Migrating to a new country can be challenging and time consuming, but the more research you do on immigration requirements while still in your home country, the smoother the process will be. Be cautious if you are using a recruiter, and gather as much information as possible on the recruitment process prior to entering the United States. This way you can reduce your risk of mistreatment and intimidation and increase the likelihood of achieving your professional goals.

RESOURCES

Anticipating Your Move to the United States

Twelve Months Left to Go

With a year still to go before a move, many people think they have plenty of time to arrange things, so they just put it off or forget about it. It is best to start the process as early as possible so that you have adequate time to put your affairs in order and to prepare for migration.

At this point in time, you should be ensuring that your passport has plenty of time left on it (usually 2 years) and checking that you have original copies of all your birth/marriage/divorce paperwork. This also should be done for anyone who may be traveling with you. If you have any outstanding debts, try to get those in order and start educating yourself on the job market of the place to which you would like to move. Check on visa policies and procedures at the U.S. Department of State Web site at http://www.travel.state.gov/visa/visa_1750.html.

Six Months Left to Go

At this point, time generally starts to move very quickly. It is a good idea to obtain quotes from shipping companies and to check flight prices so that you can get the best deals, especially if you are paying for the flight yourself. If you can, open a bank account in the United States. Because official paperwork can often take a while, you should at this point ask your bank for credit references. Also, ask your dentist and doctor for your records so that you can take these with you when you sign up with new health care professionals in the United States. Check on immunizations that you will need before entering the United States, and develop a time table for receiving them. Make sure that you have a copy of your immunizations to take with you. For a list of immunizations for U.S. immigration, check the Department of State Web site at http://travel.state.gov/visa/immigrants/info/info_1331.html.

Two Months to Go

At this stage, you will find that most of your time is spent thinking about moving or organizing the move. If you are responsible for making living arrangements in the United States, they should be in progress now. If you will be traveling with children, see if you can register them for their new schools and make sure they have all their friends' contact information to take with them. Start saying goodbye to friends now as time will run out quickly.

One Month to Go

With only 1 month left to go, you need to ensure that you have informed all the official agencies, such as the postal service, and service providers, such as telephone companies, of your move. You should start packing any nonessential items and ensure that you have all your important paperwork in a small travel file. This will make your life much easier when you are searching for things on arrival. Also, start transferring money to your foreign bank account so it is there when you arrive.

One Week to Go

At this stage, everything should be finalized, and you should be getting excited about your new venture in life. Cancel any newspaper subscriptions or milk deliveries, and if you have sold your car, cancel the insurance on it. Make sure that your goods are already shipped, and get rid of anything else that you don't need. Set aside some time to spend with friends and family as you will miss them when you are gone. If you want to have local currency when you arrive in the United States, buy some of that. Make sure that you have copies of your travelers' check numbers, insurance policy numbers, passport, and visa documents in a separate and safe place in case they are lost or stolen. As an added precaution, leave copies with family or friends.

Saying Goodbye

Make sure you leave plenty of time to say goodbye to people, and plan how you will keep in contact with them. Remember that in the first few weeks you will be very busy settling in so be realistic about how often you will make contact so that your friends and family will not worry about you. It is helpful to obtain contact information for all those people close to you. There will be times when you can not find your address book or the paper on which you wrote the information. Put all the information on your computer, if you have one, on a computer disc or wand that you can take with you, or in a file with the rest of your important paperwork.

REFERENCES

AcademyHealth. (2008). *Voluntary code of ethical conduct for the recruitment of foreign-educated nurses to the United States.* Retrieved April 24, 2009, from http://www.fair internationalrecruitment.org/TheCode.pdf

Brush, B., Sochalski, J., & Berger, A. (2004). Imported care: Recruiting foreign nurses to U.S. health care facilities. *Health Affairs, 23*(3), 78–87.

The Commission on Graduates of Foreign Nursing Schools. (2002). *Characteristics of foreign nurse graduates in the United States workforce.* Philadelphia: Author.

The Commission on Graduates of Foreign Nursing Schools. (2005). *Survey of employers of foreign-educated nurses.* Unpublished research study.

The Commission on Graduates of Foreign Nursing Schools. (2007). *Trends in international nurse migration.* Unpublished research study.

The Commission on Graduates of Foreign Nursing Schools. (2008). *Group moves to prevent unethical recruitment of foreign-educated nurses.* Special Notices and Alerts, December 2008. Philadelphia: Author.

The Commission on Graduates of Foreign Nursing Schools & AcademyHealth. (2007). *Focus group report on international nurse recruitment.* Unpublished report.

Department of Health and Human Services. (2002). *Projected supply, demand and shortages of registered nurses: 2000–2020.* Retrieved April 29, 2009, from http://bhpr. hrsa.gov/nursing/

Focus Migration. (2006). *Remittances—A bridge between migration and development.* Retrieved February 10, 2009, from http://www.focusmigration.de/uploads/tx_wil pubdb/PB05_Remit.pdf

International Council of Nurses. (2007). *Position statement: Ethical nurse recruitment.* Retrieved February 12, 2009, from http://www.icn.ch/psrecruit01.htm

Kingma, M. (2006). *Nurses on the move.* Ithaca, NY: Cornell University Press.

Pittman, P., Folsom, A., Bass, E., & Leonhardy, K. (2007). *U.S. based international nurse recruitment: Structure and practices of a burgeoning industry.* Washington, DC: AcademyHealth.

Seago, J. (2008). *The global nursing shortage and nurse migration.* Retrieved February 10, 2009, from http://www.cpath.org/sitebuildercontent/sitebuilderfiles/seago_nurse_ migration_slides.ppt

3

Entry Into the United States

DONNA R. RICHARDSON
CATHERINE R. DAVIS

In This Chapter

Immigration: Entering the United States

Occupational Visas

Applying for a Visa

Practical Nurses and Visas

Immigration Requirements for Nurses

The VisaScreen Program

The VisaScreen Process

Summary

Keywords

Affidavit: A sworn statement or written declaration made in the presence of someone authorized to administer pledges.

Associate degree: A degree earned on completion of a 2-year program of study at a community college, junior college, technical school, or other institution of higher education.

Asylum status: Protection and immunity from extradition granted by a government to a foreign political refugee.

Attestation: The action of stating that something is true, especially in a formal written statement.

Backlog: A quantity of unfinished business or work that has built up over a period of time and must be dealt with before progress can be made.

Compliance: Readiness to conform or agree to do something; a state in which someone or something is in accordance with established guidelines, specifications, or legislation.

Consular: Having to do with a consul, an official appointed by a government to reside in a foreign country to represent the commercial interests of foreign citizens who come from the official's home country.

Endorsement: Acceptance by one U.S. state of a professional license issued to an individual by another U.S. state or jurisdiction.

Petition: An appeal to or request made of a higher authority.

Refugee status: Protection granted by a government to someone who has fled another country, often because of political oppression or persecution.

Retribution: Something meted out or given to someone as punishment for something he or she has done.

Retrogression: The procedural delay in issuing an immigrant visa when there are more people applying for immigrant visas in a given year than the total number of visas available.

Test of nursing knowledge: An examination that tests understanding of the major areas of nursing (adult health nursing, nursing of children, maternal/infant nursing, and psychiatric/mental health nursing), critical thinking ability, and ability to apply nursing principles to the clinical situation.

Third-party authorization: Occurs when the individual for whose benefit a contract is created gives another person the right to act on that individual's behalf.

Unencumbered: Not held back or delayed because of difficulties or problems, for example, a nursing license that is not revoked, suspended, or made probationary or conditional by a licensing or regulatory authority as a result of disciplinary action.

A nurse who plans to enter the United States to practice nursing will have to satisfy requirements set by both immigration and licensing agencies. These include requirements that have been established for entry into the United States and for practicing nursing in one or more states within the United States. This chapter will discuss the various immigration processes required of a foreign-educated nurse who wishes to enter the United States to practice as a licensed practical/vocational nurse (LPN/LVN) or as a registered nurse (RN).

IMMIGRATION: ENTERING THE UNITED STATES

Immigration requirements establish the conditions that noncitizens must meet in order to enter the United States. A nurse who wishes to enter the United States to work will encounter three main U.S. federal agencies involved in the immigration process. The U.S. Citizenship and Immigration Services (USCIS) is an agency within the U.S. Department of Homeland Security (DHS) that is responsible for processing immigrant visa applications and **petitions** for occupational visas. The U.S. Department of Labor (DOL) is responsible for processing labor certifications. A labor certification is a document filed by a U.S. employer that demonstrates a lack of U.S. nurses available to fill a vacant nursing position. Finally, the U.S. Department of State (DOS) is responsible for granting the visa upon receipt of all required documents, fingerprints, and medical and background checks. A listing of common visa terms and their meanings as well as frequently asked questions about admission to the United States are included in Appendix B.

Selecting a Visa Type

The type of visa you must apply for depends on whether you are attempting to enter the United States to work, study, visit, or join family. Requirements differ based on your desired length of stay and your country of origin. There are several types of visas that provide nurses entry into the United States. The majority of nurses enter the United States on occupational or work visas. Others arrive as spouses or family members of immigrants who are now residents of the United States. Some have married U.S. citizens. Table 3.1 outlines the types of U.S. visas available to nurses.

Visa Issues

As you consider applying for a visa, be aware that requests for visas from some countries, for example, the Philippines, China, and India, always exceed the yearly quota. It may, therefore, take up to 14 years for that applicant's visa number to be called. Similar delays also occur for family visas, that is, when the visa holder has parents or siblings who will come later or when the spouse and minor children do not accompany the immigrant.

There are quotas for visas. Each country is allowed a certain number of visas per year. Each visa category also has a limited number of visas. Once the country quota is reached, no more visas can be processed until the next year. Up until 2005, there were usually about 20,000 visas left over each year because of the USCIS **backlog.** That has not been the case since 2005, when the USCIS became more streamlined and was able to process visa applications more efficiently, leading to what is called **retrogression.**

Retrogression

Retrogression is the procedural delay in issuing visas when more visa applications have been received than visa slots exist. The DOS determines when it is necessary to impose limits on the allocation of immigrant visa numbers. They also determine to which countries retrogression will apply.

Table 3.1

OCCUPATIONAL VISAS AND IMMIGRATION OPTIONS FOR NURSES AND ALLIED HEALTH CARE WORKERS

VISA TYPE/ CLASSIFICATION	CATEGORY	WHO QUALIFIES	DESCRIPTION
Green Card	Permanent	RNs, LPNs, Physical Therapists, Occupational Therapists, Medical Technologists, Medical Technicians, Speech-Language Pathologists, Audiologists, and Physician Assistants	Foreign health care workers may qualify for a permanent visa through various processes. Registered nurses and physical therapists may qualify under a process known as Schedule A designation, while others will need to go through the labor certification.
H-1B Visa	Temporary	Physical Therapists, Occupational Therapists, Medical Technologists, Speech-Language Pathologists, Audiologists, Physician Assistants, and RNs with a bachelor's degree working in a nursing job that requires a bachelor or higher degree	Allows a foreign national to work in a position that requires at least a bachelor's degree. There are two criteria for an H-1B visa: (1) the position must require at least a bachelor's degree; and (2) the foreign worker must have at least a bachelor's degree.
H-1C Visa	Temporary	RNs	Created in 1999 when Congress passed the Nursing Relief for Disadvantaged Areas Act. It applies only to health care facilities in medically disadvantaged areas. The Act was renewed in 2006.
TN Status	Temporary (Renewable)	Canadian or Mexican: RNs, Physical Therapists, Occupational Therapists, and Medical Technologists	The North American Free Trade Agreement (NAFTA) allows employers to hire Canadian or Mexican citizens to work in the United States under a streamlined process.
F-1	Temporary (Renewable)	Students such as those attending RN-to-BSN programs	Eligible to adjust to H-1B or permanent status after completion of education.

Under retrogression, visa applications are not processed until the backlog is completed. Retrogression may be limited to immigrants from select countries or from all countries. In 2004, when retrogression was ordered, it only applied to China, India, and the Philippines and lasted for several months. Retrogression again was declared in November 2006 for all countries and continues to the present, effectively causing a major decrease in the recruitment and certification of foreign-educated nurses.

OCCUPATIONAL VISAS

Occupational visas require an employer sponsor and **compliance** with the labor certification process. Occupational visas can be permanent or temporary.

A permanent visa allows an immigrant to stay in the United States indefinitely. A permanent visa recipient is granted a permanent resident card, commonly called a *green card.* Although it has not actually been green since 1964, the permanent resident card is still universally referred to as a "green card." You can retain legal permanent resident status as long as you do not leave the United States for longer than a year without a reentry permit. The green card must be renewed every 10 years. Registered nurses and licensed practical nurses (LPNs) are eligible for a green card.

A temporary visa limits the amount of time a nurse can stay in the United States. Those who enter the country on temporary visas are considered nonimmigrants. Temporary occupational visas are not available to everyone. Registered nurses are eligible for the following temporary (nonimmigrant) visas: Trade NAFTA (TN) status, H-1B, and H-1C. They also may qualify for student or training visas, which may allow nurses to work limited hours.

Trade NAFTA Status

Trade NAFTA (TN) status is available only to nurses from Canada or Mexico. The North American Free Trade Agreement (NAFTA) eased restrictions on the immigration of workers and importation of products among the United States, Canada, and Mexico. Registered nurses are one of several groups of workers who can enter the United States with TN status. The nurse must be a citizen of either Canada or Mexico, must have a written job offer from a U.S. employer, and must hold a nursing license in Canada or Mexico as well as in the U.S. state of intended practice.

Nurses who immigrated to either Canada or Mexico and became citizens of those countries are eligible for TN status if they meet the qualifications listed previously. For example, many nurses from Canada who are in the United States on TN status were born in India, Jamaica, the Philippines, or the United Kingdom.

Duration of Trade NAFTA Status

Initially, TN status duration was for a 1-year period and required annual renewal. However, on October 16, 2008, the Department of Homeland Security announced that TN status would be extended for up to 3 years. The number of renewals that a nurse may apply for is currently unlimited, although some immigration opponents believe that renewal of TN status should be limited and should not be used as a permanent form of temporary status. A benefit of TN status is that it is not affected by external factors such as retrogression.

Canadian Nurses

The majority of nurses holding TN status are from Canada and are not required to have a visa to enter the United States. Many TN nurses commute between Canada and the states of Michigan, Maine, and Minnesota on a daily basis. The Canadian nurse who is coming into the United States only needs to show proof of his/her citizenship, a letter of intended employment, the required licenses, and the VisaScreen certificate at the Canadian port of entry, which can be at a border crossing or an airport. The process can be completed in less than 1 day.

Mexican Nurses

The TN process for Mexican nurses is more complex and requires a visa and **consular** processing. The employer must file a labor certification and an I-129 petition for nonimmigrant workers. The process can take a day or up to a week. The educational comparability requirement has been difficult to meet for Mexican-educated nurses because nurse educators in the United States and Canada consider the majority of nursing education programs in Mexico to be at the vocational level.

Since 2005, CGFNS and the International Bilingual Nurses Alliance have worked with the Mexican nursing community, the Mexican consulate, the Mexican Overseas Program, and the Secretaría de Educación Pública (SEP; Public Education Secretariat) to develop consistent nursing education standards and ensure licensure validation processes in order to minimize the challenges for Mexican nurses who wish to migrate. Mexican nurses also have the challenge of English language proficiency, which is generally not an issue for Canadians entering under TN status.

The H-1B Nonimmigrant Visa

The H-1B is a temporary or nonimmigrant visa that is given for a 3-year term, after which it can be extended for an additional 3 years. H-1B visas require that the individual hold a baccalaureate degree, and they are available only for individuals who have been recruited for employment that requires a minimum of a baccalaureate degree for an entry-level position. The majority of foreign-educated nurses do not qualify for an H-1B visa because most entry-level nursing positions in the United States are open to nurses who hold diplomas, **associate degrees,** or baccalaureates in nursing. However, foreign-educated nurses are eligible for an H-1B visa if they are filling positions that require a baccalaureate or higher degree, such as supervisory or faculty positions.

Qualifying for an H-1B Visa

Advanced practice nurses (nurse practitioners, certified nurse anesthetists, clinical nurse specialists, and certified nurse midwives) also qualify for H-1B visas because in the United States these roles require post-baccalaureate or master's education. Critical care nurses and operating room nurses also may qualify for H-1B visas if they meet minimum experience requirements and have attained professional certification by U.S.-recognized certifying organizations for the specialty.

Some employers have given titles and advertised jobs as needing more education and skills than a typical staff nurse when the job was, in fact, a general staff position. The Department of Homeland Security issued a memorandum in 2002 and Employer Information Bulletin 19 in December 2004 describing which nursing jobs qualify for H-1B positions (see Appendix B). The USCIS has withdrawn H-1B visas granted to nurses who were subsequently found to be in general staff positions.

Another potential issue with H-1B visas is that the number is currently limited to 65,000 per year. Furthermore, nurses must compete with other professionals, including engineers and computer specialists, for those limited visa slots. In the last 2 years, when the visa process opened on April 1, the quota was filled within 3 days. All excess applications over the quota were returned to the applicants. Those eligible were chosen by lottery. An exemption from the visa cap is available for employers who employ nurses in higher education institutions, nonprofit entities affiliated to institutions of higher education, or nonprofit or governmental research organizations.

In 2009 the H-1B visa quota was not filled for more than a month because global economic instability had resulted in employers curtailing recruitment of foreign-educated workers. This opened additional slots for allied health care professionals eligible for H-1B visas, such as physical therapists.

The H-1C Nonimmigrant Visa

The Nursing Relief for Disadvantaged Areas Act (NRDAA) of 1999 designated this temporary visa, the H-1C, for RNs only. It is limited to a total of 500 nurses per year and then only to 25 nurses for each state that qualifies. The nurse can only be recruited by certain hospitals in areas that have been determined by the U.S. Department of Health and Human Services (HHS) to have a critical shortage of health care workers. These facilities must have specific, minimum percentages of Medicare and Medicaid patients (35% and 28%, respectively) and have no less than 190 licensed acute care beds (8 CFR 214.2(h) (1)(ii)). Medicare is the U.S. government health plan for the elderly and permanently disabled. Medicaid is the U.S. government health plan for individuals and families with low income and resources.

The original H-1C visa was for 3 years and could not be renewed. The category expired June 13, 2005. However, Congress granted an extension in December 2006 that ends December 20, 2009. During its first 5 years, no more than 150 nurses were granted H-1C visas each year because so few hospitals met the requirements.

The H-1A Nonimmigrant Visa

In 1989, the Immigration Nursing Relief Act (INRA) provided the temporary H-1A visa for RNs. There were no caps (limits) placed on the number of nurses admitted under the temporary H-1A visa, which was given for a period of 5 years. The H-1A visa category expired on September 1, 1995; however, H-1A nurses current as of October 11, 1996, were extended until September 30, 1997. Many believe this visa category was ended due to a miscalculation that there was no longer a significant shortage of nurses. There have been several attempts to resurrect the H-1A visa, but the U.S. Congress has rejected those efforts.

Student Visas

Those who are in the United States on student or training visas must apply to adjust to another status if they wish to stay in the United States either temporarily or permanently upon completion of the education program. Because those actions must be done within a limited time period, it is important for the nurse to consult his/her immigration attorney or the academic institution's Office of International Students for advice regarding the adjustment process.

APPLYING FOR A VISA

The first step in applying for a visa is filling out the petition for immigration, an I-140 form. Registered nurses are considered "skilled workers"—based on 2 years of post-secondary education—as well as professionals, which makes them eligible for employment-based *Third Preference* visas. Third Preference visas are for skilled workers capable of performing a job requiring at least 2 years training or experience; professionals with a baccalaureate degree, or members of a profession with at least a university bachelor's degree; and other workers capable of filling positions requiring less than 2 years training or experience.

Visa Application Documents

In addition to an I-140 form and the required fees, the employer and employee must submit the following necessary documents: a statement of valid prevailing wage; copies of all in-house media, such as printed and electronic job advertisements; a VisaScreen certificate from CGFNS International; the CGFNS Certification Program (CP) certificate, or a U.S. nursing license, or a letter confirming passage of the NCLEX examination; a nursing diploma or degree; a nursing license from the country of education, if held; nursing school transcripts; a marriage certificate, if married; and divorce decrees, if divorced.

Schedule A—Registered Nurses

Occupations listed under Schedule A have a streamlined labor certification process. The Secretary of the DOL has determined that these occupations do not have sufficient, qualified, willing, and available U.S. workers and that similarly employed U.S. workers will not have their wages and working conditions adversely affected by the employment of immigrants. Historically, RNs have been listed under Schedule A because of a continual shortage of RNs in the United States. Due to retrogression, however, there have been no available Schedule A visas beginning October 2006 and continuing to the present. Immigration advocates have proposed expanding the quotas under Schedule A or removing them totally.

Labor Certification

The labor certification process is a mandatory requirement of employers, such as hospitals, who wish to hire foreign-educated nurses.

The process was designed to assure the public that U.S. jobs would not be given to foreign workers without well-documented proof of a shortage of U.S. workers in a particular field. Employers must submit a labor certification for each nurse they recruit from abroad. The Department of Labor requires that a notice regarding the job for which the nurse is being recruited be posted at the site of intended employment for at least 10 business days. The posting must list the prevailing wage and the job requirements. A wage survey must be completed, and the employer must also show proof of the ability to pay the wages (20 CFR 656.10Ld).

Visa Process

The time to complete the immigration process is not predictable. It varies from country to country and is affected by your ability to obtain all required documents. Another factor that influences the process is the time it takes you to successfully complete the CGFNS Certification Program, pass the NCLEX examination, and obtain the required scores on the English-language proficiency exams. All of these documents are needed to support your application for the VisaScreen certificate, which must be submitted at your visa interview.

You will need to complete the process to obtain the CGFNS certification program (CP) certificate or to pass the NCLEX examination before applying for a visa. In more than 24 states the CP certificate is a prerequisite for taking the NCLEX-RN examination. For other states, you must have completed a comprehensive educational evaluation. Both of these require that the documents come directly from the nursing school or licensing authority (primary sources) to CGFNS, the State Board of Nursing, or another credentialing organization.

Employee Sponsor

An applicant for a permanent occupational visa needs an employer sponsor. The sponsor must file the Form I-140, Petition for Alien Worker. Different forms are required for other visa categories. The form must be filed at the United States Citizenship and Immigration Service (USCIS) Service Center.

To file an I-140 form the employer must have certain documents. You must submit your nursing diploma, nursing school transcripts, nursing license from your country of education, proof of passing the NCLEX examination or a CGFNS certificate, and a copy of your passport.

Visa Petition

The employer and or immigration attorney will request the required documentation for the labor certification required by the Department of Labor (DOL). That information must document the employer's intent to hire foreign-educated nurses and its financial status. The DOL grants the labor certification application (LCA).

Once the labor certification has been granted, the visa petition is filed. USCIS will approve the petition and send it to the National Visa Center (NVC) at Portsmouth, New Hampshire. The NVC will assign you a case number and fees will be requested and must be submitted to NVC.

Visa Interview

Depending on the country in which you are located, you may be able to submit copies of your documents but, generally, the NVC requires originals. You will receive an Interview Notice from the U.S. Embassy at which you applied.

You must submit all required forms at the visa interview. This includes the medical examination report. Embassy staff will conduct the interview and will inform you if your visa is approved. If you lack required documents, then the petition will be denied and you will be given a Request for Evidence (RFE) and a time frame in which the required documents must be submitted to USCIS.

If approved, you will receive your passport with immigrant visa stamps. The visa must be used within 6 months. The passport and other documents from the embassy must be provided to U.S. immigration at the airport or border. You must carry your green card with you at all times.

Adjustment of Visa Status

When nurses seek to change their visa from temporary to permanent, they must request an adjustment of status. If the time limit on a foreign-educated nurse's temporary occupational visa expires, then the nurse must return home, or adjust his/her visa status to permanent. A nurse who came to the United States on a temporary visa in order to take the NCLEX or CGFNS examination may decide to request a permanent visa in a different category. When contemplating such changes, you should consult with an immigration attorney. If filing for an adjustment is not timely or is procedurally in error, you might lose your visa and have to return home.

PRACTICAL NURSES AND VISAS

Practical nurses are now being targeted by foreign recruiters. CGFNS has seen an exponential increase in applications for Credentials Evaluation Service (CES) reports and VisaScreen certificates by those identifying themselves as practical nurses.

Practical Nurse Education Programs

Historically, most countries outside the United States do not have practical nursing programs. CGFNS's experience has demonstrated that many foreign-educated nurses who apply as RNs are in fact educated at the secondary (vocational) level, and would be considered a practical nurse in the United States. This determination was made by evaluating the comparability of the nurse's education to that of an entry level RN in the United States. Few practical nurses have entered the United States with occupational visas because of the immigration requirements and the complex and labor-intensive process required by employers.

International advertisements for practical nurse education programs cite the need for LPNs in the United States for long-term care and home health employment. Many acute-care facilities are not recruiting LPNs, but long-term care facilities are recruiting. In fact, the long-term care industry has indicated that it has 100,000 vacancies for nursing personnel. However, only 20,000 of those vacancies are designated for RNs.

Immigration Processes for Practical Nurses

Although there is a documented need for LPNs in the United States, the immigration process is not as streamlined for LPNs as it is for RNs. Employers who wish to recruit LPNs must file a petition with the USCIS. This petition must be supported by the employer's documentation of the need for a non-U.S. worker, evidence of unsuccessful recruitment, establishment of the prevailing wage, evidence of the employer's ability to pay, necessary proof of licensure, and required notices at the worksite as part of the employer's labor certification to the DOL. Upon approval of the labor certification, USCIS can proceed with processing the visa application. The labor certification process can take up to 5 years.

Immigration Challenges for Practical Nurses

A challenge for practical nurse migration is that USCIS regulations have designated that a "professional" is an individual who has more than 2 years of education. Because practical nurse education programs tend to be less than 2 years in length, practical nurses are not considered professionals by USCIS. This means that practical nurses are not eligible for H-1B or TN temporary visas, nor do they qualify under Schedule A. Several recruitment agencies have petitioned to have LPNs included under Schedule A, but they have not been successful thus far.

Another challenge is that there is no practical nurse predictor exam like the CGFNS Qualifying Exam (Certification Program) for RNs. This means that practical nurses and their employers are not able to assess their eligibility for the NCLEX-PN examination and the likelihood of passing that examination. It also means that practical nurses are limited to 11 countries in which they can take the NCLEX-PN examination. Therefore, applicants who do not live in those 11 countries would have to travel to the closest test sites. Most employers are hesitant to accept that expense when there is no assurance that the practical nurse will be successful on the NCLEX-PN examination.

Recognition of Practical Nursing Programs

The major issue for foreign-educated practical nurses seeking entry and licensure in the United States is whether or not practical nursing is recognized as an occupation by their country of education. Some U.S. State Boards of Nursing require that a country recognize practical nursing by granting it licensure or registration in order for the practical nurse to be eligible for licensure in the United States. They also believe that a scope of practice, universal standards of education, practice standards, and disciplinary or oversight processes developed by the nursing authority must exist for the occupation. Many assert that there is no demonstrable quality control of nursing programs or practice without such processes.

Other State Boards of Nursing believe that if a practical nurse can pass the NCLEX-PN examination after completing a comparable education program, then his/her minimum competency has been demonstrated. Those states do not require licensure/registration in the country of education. It appears that foreign-educated practical nurses may seek licensure in gateway states (entry states), intending to work elsewhere once licensed. Practical nurses who have passed the NCLEX-PN examination in such states have unfortunately been denied licensure by **endorsement** in some states.

If you are a practical nurse seeking U.S. licensure, you should check with the State Board of Nursing in your intended state of practice so that you are aware of the requirements for licensure in that state.

IMMIGRATION REQUIREMENTS FOR NURSES

Section 343 of the 1996 Illegal Immigration Reform and Immigrant Responsibility Act (IIRIRA) mandated that health care professionals not born or educated in the United States must undergo a federal screening program in order to receive an occupational visa. Section 343 authorized CGFNS, through its division the International Commission on Healthcare Professions (ICHP), to conduct such a program by verifying and evaluating the educational and licensure credentials of RNs and LPNs as well as seven other categories of health care professionals: physical therapists, occupational therapists, audiologists, speech-language pathologists, medical technologists, medical technicians, and physician assistants. CGFNS designated this process as VisaScreen: Visa Credentials Assessment.

Section 343 Screening

Section 343 screening includes: an assessment of the individual's education to ensure that it is comparable to that of a U.S. graduate in the same profession; verification that licenses are valid and **unencumbered;** demonstration of written and oral English language proficiency; and, in the case of RNs, verification that the nurse has either passed the CGFNS Qualifying Exam or passed the NCLEX-RN examination.

English Language Proficiency Examinations

The English language proficiency examinations and their required scores are mandated in the 2003 Final Regulations implementing Section 343 of IIRIRA. The nurse must demonstrate competency in oral and written English on English tests approved by the U.S. Departments of Education and Health and Human Services as recommended to the Department of Homeland Security (DHS). Nurses must take either: (1) the Test of English as a Foreign Language (TOEFL), plus the Test of Written English (TWE) and Test of Spoken English (TSE); or (2) the TOEFL iBT (Internet-based TOEFL); or (3) the Test of English for International Communication (TOEIC), plus TSE and TWE; or (4) the International English Language Testing System (IELTS). English test scores are valid for 2 years, so they must be current when all other required VisaScreen documentation has been received. Scores from the ETS tests (TOEFL, TWE, TSE, iBT, and TOEIC) and the IELTS examinations cannot be interchanged. See Table 3.2 for the required English scores by profession. Nurses educated in designated English-speaking countries are exempt from this requirement.

Table 3.2

SECTION 343 ENGLISH LANGUAGE SCORE REQUIREMENTS BY PROFESSION

Health Care Profession	ETS OPTION 1*			ETS OPTION 2*			ETS OPTION 3*		IELTS OPTION 4	
	TOEFL Test of English As A Foreign Language	TWE Test of Written English	TSE Test of Spoken English	TOEIC Test of English for International Communication *Listening and Reading Test*	TWE Test of Written English	TSE Test of Spoken English	TOEFL iBT Test of English as a Foreign Language Internet-Based Test *Total*	TOEFL iBT Test of English as a Foreign Language Internet-Based Test *Speaking Section*	IELTS International English Language Testing System *Overall*	IELTS International English Language Testing System *Spoken Band*
Registered Nurse	207 (540*)	4.0	50	725	4.0	50	83	26	6.5 (Academic)	7
Practical/ Vocational Nurse	197 (530*)	4.0	50	700	4.0	50	79	26	6.0 (General) or 6.0 (Academic)	7
Physical Therapist	220 (560*)	4.5	50	—	—	—	89	26	—	—
Occupational Therapist	220 (560*)	4.5	50	—	—	—	89	26	—	—

Speech-Language Pathologist	207 (540*)	4.0	50	725	4.0	50	83	26	6.5 (Academic)	7
Audiologist	207 (540*)	4.0	50	725	4.0	50	83	26	6.5 (Academic)	7
Clinical Laboratory Scientist (Medical Technologist)	207 (540*)	4.0	50	725	4.0	50	83	26	6.5 (Academic)	7
Clinical Laboratory Technician (Medical Technician)	197 (530*)	4.0	50	700	4.0	50	79	26	6.0 (General) or 6.0 (Academic)	7
Physician Assistant	207 (540*)	4.0	50	725	4.0	50	83	26	6.5 (Academic)	7

ETS (Educational Testing Service) administers the tests shown in Options 1, 2, and 3.
Note: Combining passing test scores from both IELTS and ETS administered tests is not acceptable.

THE VISASCREEN PROGRAM

The VisaScreen program comprises four elements: educational analysis, licensure validation, English language proficiency assessment, and, in the case of RNs, examination of nursing knowledge.

The *educational analysis* ensures that the applicant's secondary and professional education meets all applicable statutory and regulatory requirements for the profession and is comparable to the education of a U.S. graduate seeking licensure. Applicants may include a photocopy of their diploma, certificate, or external examination certificate from their secondary school and nonprofessional, post-secondary school with their application. However, transcripts of professional education must come directly to CGFNS from the academic institution.

Applicants submit a *Request for Academic Records* form to each school listed in the Professional Education section of the VisaScreen application. The applicant must have completed a secondary school education that was separate from the nursing education; graduated from a government-approved, general nursing program (for RNs the program must be at least 2 years in length); and received a minimum number of hours of theoretical instruction and clinical practice in nursing care of the adult, nursing of children, maternal/infant nursing, and psychiatric/mental health nursing.

The *licensure review* evaluates all professional licenses to ensure that they are valid and unencumbered. Applicants submit a *Request for Validation of Registration/Licensure* form to the licensing/registration authorities in their country of education and in all other jurisdictions in which they have ever been licensed, whether current or expired. When the country does not have a licensure system, the individual's diploma grants the right to practice in that country and is validated as such for VisaScreen purposes. CGFNS validates all licenses, past and present, to ensure that they have not been revoked or suspended.

The *English language proficiency assessment* confirms that the applicant has demonstrated the required competency in oral and written English by submitting scores on tests approved by the U.S. Departments of Education and Health and Human Services as described previously.

Registered nurse VisaScreen applicants must pass a **test of nursing knowledge**, either the CGFNS Qualifying Exam or the NCLEX-RN examination.

Once the applicant has successfully completed all elements of the VisaScreen program, the applicant is awarded a VisaScreen certificate, which must be presented to a consular office or, in the case of adjustment of status, the attorney general as part of the visa application. Trade NAFTA applicants must present their VisaScreen certificate at the port of entry into the United States or to border agents.

VisaScreen Documents

Documents and test scores required for VisaScreen also may be required by State Boards of Nursing for licensure as well as by the DHS for immigration. Because CGFNS must receive these documents directly from the school and licensing authority in the nurse's country of education, processing times may vary; processing cannot occur until all required documents have been received. CGFNS is mindful of deadlines for immigration and licensing application purposes and works with nurses to facilitate the necessary VisaScreen processing to meet applicant deadlines. Most countries and schools assess fees for licensure validation and transcripts. The fees vary from a few dollars to more than $100. They also may charge mailing and stamp fees.

THE VISASCREEN PROCESS

In addition to all the documents that must be submitted to support the employee's petition with the employer's labor certification, there are extensive documentation requirements that must be met in order to obtain your VisaScreen certificate. This certificate is required by the USCIS in order to meet all visa requirements during your appointment at the consulate or U.S. embassy.

Beginning the Process

The VisaScreen process should be started as soon as the nurse begins to consider coming to the United States. The nurse should contact

CGFNS International, preferably via the Web, at http://www.cgfns. org. Written correspondence can be mailed to 3600 Market Street, Suite 400, Philadelphia, PA 19104. Telephone assistance is available from 8:00 A.M.–12 P.M. (EST) at (215) 349-8767.

Application Form and Handbook

The VisaScreen application and handbook are available online. To avoid confusion and mistakes in the application process, you should read all instructions and the handbook before filling out any forms. Inconsistent information will result in processing delays. All inconsistencies require written confirmation by the issuing agency as well as written clarification by the applicant.

Source Documents

Because all transcripts and licensure validations must come directly to CGFNS from the schools of nursing and licensing authorities, you must submit a request to those agencies authorizing them to release your information to CGFNS. You are responsible for paying any processing fees, taxes, or postage fees related to the application. You should request all necessary documents as soon as possible when applying for VisaScreen because the submitting agency's response can be affected by its staffing, computerization and budget capabilities.

The submitting agencies also should be advised that you might be required to have the same documents sent to several different places because the State Boards of Nursing, employers, and USCIS do not share documents. Confidentiality and privacy laws may prohibit information from being exchanged between agencies or with nongovernmental bodies.

International Mail

To ensure timely delivery of documents to CGFNS, you should provide a prepaid, preaddressed envelope to the submitting agencies for the documents to be sent to CGFNS. Remember, the documents must come directly from the agency to CGFNS. Documents that are sent by a third party, such as you as the applicant or a recruiter, will *not* be considered.

Always be sure to use a mail or courier service that provides a tracking number, such as FedEx or UPS, when submitting important documents to CGFNS. Traceable mail alleviates the stress of locating mail that cannot be matched to applications and confirms that the documents have been sent and received.

Preventing Processing Delays

Common reasons for delays in processing include incomplete information, missing signatures, inconsistent information between the documents and the application, and expired documents. Licenses must be validated by the issuing agency if more than 3 years old. This is required even when licenses are deemed lifetime to ensure that no adverse incidents have affected the nurse's right to practice. All English scores must have been achieved within 2 years of the receipt of all required VisaScreen documents.

One way that you can decrease the processing time for your Visa-Screen application is by making sure that you identify all the names you have ever used, including unmarried (maiden) names and names from previous marriages, if any, when completing the application form. All name changes should be accompanied by verifying documents, such as birth certificates, marriage licenses, and divorce decrees.

Completing the Application Correctly

Dates are critical. Double check dates of school attendance, graduation, and date of birth. Remember to write out the name of the months. The European and U.S. styles of using numerical dates are different, which can cause confusion. If you are aware of date conflicts in any of your documents, provide a written explanation (**affidavit**).

When providing information on your education, give the name of all schools attended, dates attended, and degrees and diplomas or certificates received. Provide the exact full name of all schools. Do not use abbreviations or initials. If your school has closed or merged with another, check with the Ministry of Health or Education—or nurse licensing authority—to find out where the school's records are now kept, and request them to be sent to CGFNS.

Using Your CGFNS Identification Number

It is helpful to include your CGFNS identification number on all documents and correspondence so that when CGFNS receives them they can be matched with your file. CGFNS has files on over 500,000 nurses and allied health professionals. In many countries, there are birth and surnames that are very common. For example, there are over 11,000 files with the name Maria Lopez in the CGFNS database. Without middle names, dates of birth, and other vital data, appropriate and timely matching of documents is difficult.

All documents are now scanned by CGFNS, and an electronic file is created. This allows examination of all your documents by those at CGFNS when inquiries are received. No information about you will be shared with anyone, including spouses, without a **third-party authorization** form signed and submitted by you. Your CGFNS file is permanent, which means that the same file and ID number is used if you subsequently apply for any additional CGFNS services.

Maintaining Document Integrity

It is important to treat all documents with the same care and integrity that you would a patient's record and documentation. Under no circumstances should you alter any information on any document.

If a mistake is made, do not cover it up, but instead, draw a strike through the mistake and initial it. Altering a document in any way may result in the sealing of your CGFNS file and an inability to apply for CGFNS services in the future.

Document Review

CGFNS procedures require that its international credentials evaluators verify all documents. The evaluators compare dates, names, and dates of birth. They verify all seals, signatures, and watermarks and also may confirm documents with the agencies.

Academic Transcripts

Schools are asked to provide full transcripts and a breakdown of the clinical and theory hours in core nursing courses to determine the comparability of your education to that of a nurse educated in the United States. When asked to provide your professional title, use the exact terminology used in your country of education and on your nursing license. Transcripts may be denied or held if the nurse did not complete his/her military or community service.

Licenses

All foreign and U.S. licenses are reviewed to ensure that they are valid and have not been revoked or suspended. Nurses should be mindful of the licensure requirements in their country of education to ensure efficient responses to their requests for licensure validations. Some countries require payment of registration fees, even retroactively, before they will provide licensure validation to CGFNS and State Boards of Nursing.

CGFNS is aware that some countries may not allow those who completed their nursing education in that country to become licensed there because they are not citizens or residents. In other countries, individuals completing their nursing education may not be able to take licensing examinations because of language-proficiency requirements. CGFNS has alternative processes for these unlicensed nurses.

VisaScreen Attestation

It is critical to answer all application form questions thoughtfully and truthfully. A VisaScreen application can be slowed, suspended, or sealed because of altered, misrepresented, or fraudulent information. The DHS relies on the VisaScreen process for immigration, therefore, nurses must take the **attestation** required on the application seriously. It also is valued by the State Boards of Nursing and employers because it ensures that the recruitment and migration of qualified nurses protects the health and safety of patients in the United States.

Refugee Status

Special procedures have been established for nurses who have official **refugee** or **asylum status**. These are individuals who have left their country to avoid persecution or requested to stay in the United States because of fear of persecution or **retribution** if they return home.

CGFNS recognizes that these nurses may not be able to request or obtain educational or licensure documents because of political restrictions and loss or destruction of documents and/or infrastructure, such as the closing of agencies and the loss of knowledge of how policies and procedures were implemented.

Alternative Processes for VisaScreen Certification

There are two alternative processes to achieve certification as a nurse for visa purposes. Paragraph 212(r) of the Immigration and Nationality Act allows an abbreviated process that exempts certain nurses from English proficiency and educational comparability requirements.

Abbreviated Certification Process (212 (r))

To be eligible for the abbreviated 212 (r) certification process the nurse must demonstrate that he or she:

1. Has a valid and unencumbered (unrestricted) nursing license in a state where he/she intends to be employed. In addition, that state must verify that the foreign licenses are authentic and unencumbered (states that satisfy this requirement are limited to Michigan, Florida, Georgia, Illinois, and New York)—and that the nurse has passed the NCLEX-RN examination;

2. Is a graduate of a nursing program in which the language of instruction was English, and that the program was located in a country designated by CGFNS (currently includes Australia, Barbados, Canada (except most of Quebec), Ireland,

Jamaica, New Zealand, South Africa, the United Kingdom, Trinidad/Tobago, and the United States) and was in operation before November 12, 1999, or that is subsequently designated by CGFNS and any equivalent organizations approved for the credentialing of nurses. Graduates of Quebec nursing programs that instruct in English and use English textbooks, such as McGill University in Montreal, Vanier College in St. Laurent, John Abbott College in Sainte Anne de Bellevue, Dawson College in Montreal, and Heritage College in Gatineau are exempt from English language proficiency testing under section 212 (r).

Streamlined Certification Process

The second alternative is the Streamlined Certification Process. U.S.-educated nurses who were born outside the United States are exempt from the educational comparability review and English language proficiency testing generally required to obtain an occupational visa.

A nurse born outside of the United States who has graduated from an entry-level program accredited by the National League for Nursing Accrediting Commission (NLNAC) or the Commission on Collegiate Nursing Education (CCNE) qualifies. The school must provide a statement verifying graduation. All licenses have to be verified as unencumbered by the issuing agency.

SUMMARY

Foreign-educated nurses must meet state licensure and immigration requirements to practice in the United States. The foreign-educated nurse's stay in the United States is determined by the type of visa for which he/she qualifies. Most foreign-educated nurses use occupational visas, which can be temporary or permanent. Special procedures have been established under Trade NAFTA for Canadian and Mexican nurses.

The VisaScreen process has been mandated by the DHS to ensure the foreign-educated nurse's educational comparability, licensure validity, and English language proficiency and to certify his/her capability to provide safe patient care in the United States. The process can be navigated more easily by accessing the CGFNS Web site (http://www.cgfns.org) and customer service materials.

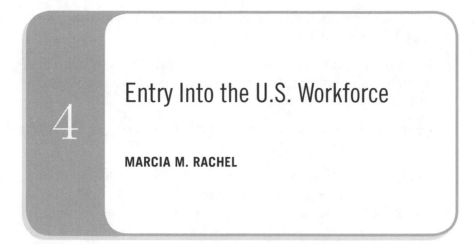

Entry Into the U.S. Workforce

MARCIA M. RACHEL

4

In This Chapter

The Philosophy of States' Rights

State Licensure Requirements

The Role of CGFNS International

The NCLEX Examinations

Summary

Keywords

Auditing: The process of reviewing, evaluating, and verifying accounts or documents, especially those of a business, organization, or institution.

Bioterrorism: Terrorism by intentional release or dissemination of biological agents, for example, bacteria, viruses, or toxins.

Criminal background check: The investigation of or search for the possibility of a person's criminal history; generally used by potential employers, lenders, and so forth, to assess the person's trustworthiness.

71

Diagnostic report: Detailed information used to identify or reflect the results of a test.

Notarized signature: A notary's stamp and signature that signifies that something, such as a signature on a legal document, is authentic and legitimate.

Peer review: An assessment of an article, piece of work, or research by experts on the subject.

Regulatory authority: A public authority or government agency responsible for enforcing standards and safety, overseeing the use of public goods and services, as well as regulating commerce; also, the power to control or direct an entity in agreement with a law or regulation.

Telenursing: Refers to the use of information technology for providing nursing services in health care.

Vocational nurse: A graduate of an accredited technical school of nursing; licensed practical nurses (LPNs) are also known as licensed vocational nurses (LVNs) in California and Texas.

Nursing licensure in the United States is at the state rather than the national level. Each state sets its own requirements for practice; thus, nurses entering the United States for purposes of employment must apply for a license in their U.S. state of intended practice. This chapter will provide detailed information on how to obtain a license to practice as a nurse in the United States.

THE PHILOSOPHY OF STATES' RIGHTS

Each U.S. state, territory, and the District of Columbia requires that an individual be legally authorized to practice as a registered nurse (RN) or licensed practical/**vocational nurse** (LPN/LVN) before being allowed to work as a nurse. LPNs are called LVNs in the states of California and Texas. Unlike most countries, the United States does not offer a single nursing license that is recognized and valid in all U.S. states and territories. Instead, each individual state has authority over nursing practice within its borders. The scope of nursing practice is defined by state laws and by regulations administered by State Boards of Nursing. These laws and regulations are known as the Nurse Practice Act, which defines the requirements for education and licensure and the responsibilities of the nurse based on the level of the individual's formal nursing education program. Nurse practice acts differ for RNs and LPNs/LVNs and vary from state to state (see chapter 7 for more information on nurse practice acts).

The principle of states' authority over matters such as regulating health care and nursing practice is often known as "states' rights." It is derived from the 10th amendment to the U.S. Constitution, which states, "the powers not delegated to the United States by the constitution, nor prohibited by it to the states, are reserved to the States respectively, or to the people" (U.S. Bill of Rights, n.d.).

States' rights, as applied to nursing, means that each state determines who does and does not practice as a nurse in that state. The only exception applies to nurses who are employed by the federal government, such as at a military base or a Veterans Administration hospital. These nurses must be licensed by at least one U.S. state or territory, whether or not they are licensed in the state in which the federal facility at which they are working is located.

Boards of Nursing

Boards of Nursing were established by state governments to protect the public's health by ensuring the safe practice of nursing. They meet this goal by establishing standards of safe nursing practice, overseeing the education of nurses, and issuing licenses to qualified applicants. They also monitor continuing compliance with the state's laws and regulations and take disciplinary action (which can include suspending or revoking licensure) against nurses who have practiced in an unsafe or incompetent manner.

Each state and territory has at least one Board of Nursing. Most states have a single Board of Nursing that regulates RNs, LPN/LVNs, and advanced practice nurses. However, four states have separate Boards of Nursing for RNs and LPN/LVNs (California, Georgia, Louisiana, and West Virginia), and one state has a separate Board for Advanced Practice Nurses (Nebraska). If you are applying for licensure in one of these states, make sure you contact the correct Board, using the application from that Board, and that you have transcripts and other documents sent to the correct address.

Composition

Boards of Nursing are government agencies that include members who are practicing nurses, nurse educators, nurse employers, and consumers. Some states have specific Board positions for physicians, advanced practice nurses, or other special groups. In addition to Board members, there are state (government) employees who work for the Board and who perform its day-to-day activities.

Role

Most Boards of Nursing are responsible for approving and regulating nursing education programs, including LPN, RN, and advanced practice nursing programs. Some Boards of Nursing also have **regulatory authority** over other health care workers such as certified nurse aides, medication technicians or assistants, dialysis technicians, and others. In other states, regulation of these workers rests with another state agency.

Boards of Nursing not only have the authority to issue licenses, but they also may revoke, suspend, or otherwise discipline a licensee if the nurse is found guilty of violating the nurse practice law.

STATE LICENSURE REQUIREMENTS

Although the principle of states' rights allows a Board of Nursing to adopt state-specific requirements that have been determined to be in the best interest of that state's citizens, most state requirements have a lot in common with each other. This section presents some general information about the licensure process, common licensure procedures, and some state-specific requirements and discusses the Nurse Licensure Compact.

Nurses may be licensed in more than one state, either by examination (for initial licensure) or through endorsement, by a State Board of Nursing, of a license issued by another state. States that have adopted the Nurse Licensure Compact allow nurses licensed in one of the states in the Compact to practice in all Compact states through mutual recognition of licensure.

When you are ready to begin the application process, you should check with the state or territory in which you wish to be licensed for the most current application and requirements. To assist you in the process, a list of resources is included at the end of this chapter.

Initial Licensure

The first nursing license issued to an individual by a U.S. state or territory is obtained by taking and passing the National Council Licensure Examination (NCLEX) and thus is referred to as licensure by examination. State Boards of Nursing set requirements regarding who is eligible for licensure by examination. These requirements include criteria such as a minimum level of education, submission of an application, payment of a fee, finger printing, and, in most cases, a **criminal background check.**

Education
Application
Fee
Immigration Requirements
Background Check
Examination

Education

LPN/LVNs educated in the United States typically attend a vocational school or community college. The course of study is generally completed in 12 to 24 months. LPN/LVN programs combine classroom lectures and supervised clinical experience, and they cover basic nursing theories, patient care, health administration, and drug administration.

Most RNs educated in the United States generally receive their initial preparation through one of three basic types of programs: associate degree, diploma, or baccalaureate.

An Associate of Arts in Nursing or Associate of Science in Nursing is generally referred to as an Associate Degree in Nursing (ADN) and requires 2 years of college-level study with a strong emphasis on clinical knowledge and skills. Most of these programs are offered in community colleges, although some are in senior colleges and universities.

Diploma in Nursing programs are 2- to 3-year programs that are offered in a hospital-based school of nursing. Graduates receive a certificate upon graduation. Few diploma programs remain in the United States, and the proportion of nurses practicing with a diploma is rapidly decreasing. Many have affiliated with a college and include some college level courses so that graduates who choose to do so may easily continue on for a baccalaureate degree.

Bachelor of Science in Nursing (BSN) programs are 4 years in length and offered in colleges and universities. They have an enhanced emphasis on leadership and research as well as clinically focused courses.

Regardless of the type of RN or LPN program the nurse attends, it must be one that is approved by the state's approving body (usually the State Board of Nursing). For foreign-educated nurses, Boards of Nursing will require either an evaluation by CGFNS or by some other credentials review company, or they will evaluate the education themselves to ensure that it is comparable to that of a U.S.-educated nurse. You should check the state's Web site regarding how that evaluation is done because the process varies widely.

Evaluation of Education. The Board of Nursing will need an official transcript from your school of nursing. This means that the transcript must come directly from the school to the Board of Nursing office. If you attended more than one school of nursing for your basic education, you should have each school send an official transcript. Many Boards will accept evaluations from CGFNS International or another credentialing service in lieu of the official transcript from the school. Check with the specific Board of Nursing to find out if this is the case.

Education
Application
Fee
Immigration Requirements
Background Check
Examination

Application

Most Boards of Nursing have the application for licensure by examination available on their Web site. You will need to download the application along with the instructions, and follow each step carefully. If there are special requirements for foreign-educated applicants, they will be stated in the instructions. Some Boards of Nursing require that you apply online.

Preventing Delays. In order to prevent any delays, be sure to print clearly or use a typewriter when you are completing the application and to complete all sections of the application. Leaving required information blank will cause the Board of Nursing to return the application to you for completion and will delay the process. The application requires that you submit a passport photo of yourself, and some require a **notarized signature.**

If your mailing address changes after you have submitted the application, notify the Board of Nursing in writing. Much communication about your application, including mailing of your actual license, requires a physical mailing address. If you are not in a permanent situation that allows you to receive mail reliably, you might want to use a family member's address until you obtain more permanent housing.

Arrests and Criminal Convictions. Most Boards of Nursing ask questions on the application about arrests and criminal convictions. It is essential that you answer these questions truthfully. If you answer "yes" to this question on the application, be prepared to supply copies of the conviction or arrest record. Answering "yes" does not automatically exclude you from being licensed, but it will involve additional review by the Board of Nursing. However, if your background check uncovers a conviction that you had not disclosed, the Board of Nursing may consider that falsification of your application, and you could be denied licensure on this basis alone.

If you already have copies of the related arrest or conviction records, you can attach them to the application when it is submitted. This will allow the Board of Nursing to begin the review as soon as they receive your application and might save you several weeks or months of time. Boards of Nursing are primarily interested in crimes against persons and crimes involving drug or alcohol use or abuse, but each state has the right to determine which types of convictions prevent an applicant from being licensed. Remember, the Board of Nursing exists to protect the public within that state from unsafe nursing practice, and their regulations and rules help them to accomplish this.

Temporary Permits. In some states, applicants for licensure by examination are offered temporary (or interim) permits that allow the applicant to practice in a supervised position and under certain circumstances until the NCLEX results have been received. This temporary permit is not automatically issued, and some states exclude foreign-educated nurses from receiving a temporary permit, so you should ask about that if you are interested. New York's Board of Nursing will issue a temporary permit for one year's duration if you hold a CGFNS Certification Program certificate.

Fitness for Practice. Some states ask questions about your fitness to practice as a nurse. This means they want to know whether there is any physical or mental impairment or other condition that would prevent you from being able to practice safely as a nurse. These questions might be about your mental or emotional status, your physical ability to practice as a nurse, or other similar issues. Again, each Board of Nursing has the authority to determine who is fit to practice within their state, while being mindful of labor laws. There are laws in the United States that protect the disabled from discrimination in hiring practices and in promotions.

Keep a copy of all applications and documents sent to a Board of Nursing. You may need to refer to parts of the application during subsequent conversations or e-mail communications with the Board of Nursing, and having a copy will be helpful to you and the Board representative.

Education
Application
Fee
Immigration Requirements
Background Check
Examination

Fee

There may be several fees associated with an application to a single Board of Nursing. First, there will be the basic application fee. In states where a background check is mandatory, you will be required to be fingerprinted, which involves another fee. If the state issues a temporary permit, that will be yet another fee. Unless the Board of Nursing specifically allows it, do not combine all fees into one payment. Instead, submit a separate payment for each fee, and make a note regarding what the payment is for.

Method of Payment. Some states will *not* accept personal checks, but most will accept payment by money order or cashier's check, and many will accept payment by credit card. Very few states, if any, will issue a refund once payment is received, so make sure you are ready to send the fee before you mail it.

If you are applying to a state that accepts personal checks, be aware that extra penalties will be imposed if you have insufficient funds in your bank account to cover the check. In addition, the Board of Nursing can cancel any license application if it was paid for by a check that did not clear the bank. To be safe, avoid using personal checks for licensure fees. In addition, *never* send cash through the mail as payment for a program or service.

Education
Application
Fee
Immigration Requirements
Background Check
Examination

Immigration Requirements

The U.S. federal government is the authority regarding all immigration issues. Individual U.S. states and territories must follow all U.S. government requirements related to issuing a license to someone who is not a U.S. citizen. You will need to obtain the proper work visa before you are allowed to enter the country, and the Board of Nursing must have proof of these documents (see chapter 3, "Immigration Requirements for Nurses"). The U.S. Citizenship and Immigration Service (USCIS) can provide information and assistance regarding this process (http://www.uscis.gov/portal/site/uscis).

Education
Application
Fee
Immigration Requirements
Background Check
Examination

Background Check

Some Boards of Nursing require a background check for all applicants. They also may require a copy of your fingerprints, which will be compared to files in various law enforcement agencies. If the Board of Nursing requires this, its application instructions will direct you to law enforcement agencies for fingerprint cards, and there will be a fee for the process.

Table 4.1

U.S. STATES REQUIRING BACKGROUND CHECK FOR LICENSURE

Alabama	Iowa	North Dakota
Alaska	Kentucky	Ohio
American Samoa	Louisiana-RN	Oklahoma
Arizona	Maryland	Rhode Island
Arkansas	Missouri	South Dakota
Florida	Nevada	Utah
Guam	New Hampshire	Washington
Hawaii	New Jersey	Wisconsin
Idaho	New Mexico	Wyoming
Illinois	North Carolina	

Finding a match between your fingerprint and law enforcement records does not necessarily mean that you will be denied licensure by the Board of Nursing. It does mean, however, that the Board of Nursing will review any conviction or arrest history and will then make a decision based on its charge to protect the public in that state. Approximately 55% of the U.S. Boards of Nursing require a criminal background check for licensure (National Council of State Boards of Nursing, Inc. [NCSBN], 2007). Table 4.1 lists the states and territories that currently require a criminal background check.

Education
Application
Fee
Immigration Requirements
Background Check
Examination

Examination

All states and most U.S. territories require that you pass the NCLEX-RN® or NCLEX-PN® examination before being licensed to practice in that state. The only exception is Puerto Rico, which does not require either NCLEX examination for licensure and offers its own examinations in both Spanish and English. Nurses who take the Puerto Rico examinations will be required to take an NCLEX examination to work in any U.S. state and in any other U.S. territory.

The NCLEX-RN and NCLEX-PN examinations are designed to test the knowledge, skills, and abilities essential to the safe and effective practice of nursing at the entry level. These tests are developed and owned by the National Council of State Boards of Nursing, Inc. (NCSBN), which administers these examinations on behalf of its member Boards, including the Boards of Nursing in all 50 states, the District of Columbia, American Samoa, Guam, the Northern Mariana Islands, and the U.S. Virgin Islands.

Examination Administration. The NCLEX examinations are provided in a computerized adaptive testing (CAT) format and are currently administered by a private company, Pearson VUE, in their network of testing centers called Pearson Professional Centers (PPC). These testing centers are located throughout the United States and in some foreign countries. Table 4.2 lists the approved countries where the NCLEX examinations are given.

The NCLEX is given only in English, and application forms and instructions are available only in English. All items are developed and validated using the expertise of practicing nurses, educators, and nursing regulators from throughout the United States. Some states also may require that you meet English language proficiency requirements. Those requirements will be on the individual Board's Web site.

In summary, as you go about the process of applying for licensure by examination in the United States, you should work through these steps:

- Decide on the state in which you will be working. You should only apply to one state at a time for licensure by examination.

Table 4.2

2009 NCLEX INTERNATIONAL TEST SITES ADMINISTERED BY PEARSON VUE

COUNTRY	CITY/PROVINCE	COUNTRY	CITY/PROVINCE
Australia	Sydney	Mexico	Mexico City
Canada	Montreal	Taiwan	Taipei
	Toronto	Japan	Chiyoda-ku
	Vancouver		Yokohama
Germany	Frankfurt	United Kingdom	London
India	Bangalore	South Korea	Seoul
	Chennai	Hong Kong	Hong Kong
	Hyderabad	Philippines	Manila
	Mumbai		
	New Delhi		

- Contact that Board (or view their Web site). Locate a copy of that Board's Nurse Practice Act online and keep it for reference.
- Request or print a copy of an application for licensure by examination as either an RN or an LPN/LVN.
- Review the application directions and talk to someone at the Board of Nursing about requirements for licensure. Ask specifically about special requirements for foreign-educated nurses.
- Meet all immigration requirements.
- Register and take the NCLEX examination.
- Notify the Board of Nursing in writing any time you change your address.

License Renewal

Nursing licenses in the United States are not lifetime documents. While states may use somewhat different procedures or terminology, nursing licenses must be periodically renewed or re-registered. Most licenses must be renewed every 2 years, but a few states renew annually, including: Connecticut, Kentucky, Louisiana RN and PN, Maryland, Washington, and West Virginia RN and PN. A few other states, Arizona, Iowa, New York, and Tennessee, renew every 3 or 4 years (NCSBN, 2007).

Most states will mail a renewal notice several weeks or months before the license expires. The renewal must be completed and returned to the Board of Nursing before the deadline in order to renew the license. However, some states are moving toward a paperless renewal system that will require the nurse to renew online using the Internet. Whether the system is by mail or online, the State Board (or other licensing agency) will review your renewal application and determine if you have met all requirements, in which case the Board can renew your license, request additional information, or deny the renewal.

Depending on the state of licensure, the renewal application may be as simple as updating the mailing address and returning a fee. Or it may be more complicated, requiring completion of a much longer form that asks questions about recent criminal convictions, work history, and continuing education activities.

Continued Competency

Some Boards of Nursing require proof of continuing competency before your license is renewed. Some require that you must have practiced as a nurse for a certain amount of time and/or within a certain period of time for renewal. Others have some combination requirements that may include **peer review,** continuing education, minimum practice hours, or some other mechanism to assess competency. Still other states have no renewal requirements specific to mandatory practice or mandatory continuing education.

Continuing Education

About 25% of U.S. Boards of Nursing require topic-specific education to obtain or renew the license. For example, the Nevada Board of Nursing has a one-time requirement for a course on **bioterrorism;** the Florida Board of Nursing requires education related to domestic violence; the Iowa Board of Nursing requires education related to child abuse; and the Ohio, Texas, and Alabama Boards of Nursing require a course that deals with nursing laws and regulation. Other topics that are required by some Boards of Nursing include end-of-life care, pain management, domestic violence, pharmacology, prevention of medication errors, and HIV/AIDS (NCSBN, 2007).

You should check with the Board of Nursing where you will be licensed to determine if they require any specific continuing education for initial licensure or for renewal of the license. Remember, Boards of Nursing have the authority to revise their regulations throughout the year as needed, so visit their Web sites on a regular basis to find out about recent changes to this requirement.

Boards of Nursing that require continuing education for renewal have established **auditing** mechanisms for the verification of what is reported to them. You might be selected as someone who will be audited for a particular period of time. If this happens, follow the directions carefully, keep copies of everything you submit, and meet the Board's deadline. You should always keep a file of certificates of completion of continuing education courses you take. In addition, you should make certain that the continuing education courses you take are approved or accredited by an approved agency for nursing continuing education.

Licensure by Endorsement

When a nurse is already licensed in one state and then applies to be licensed in an additional state, it is called licensure by endorsement. In this case, the second state does not require you to take an additional licensure examination. Instead, that state recognizes the passing result on the original NCLEX examination and, if you meet all other requirements, allows you to be licensed. Many people incorrectly call this process *reciprocity,* but the State Boards uniformly refer to it as endorsement.

Completing the Application Process

You must still submit an application, pay a fee, send transcripts or meet the credentials review requirements, and meet any other requirements of the Board of Nursing to be licensed by endorsement. For example, some states will require a background and/or fingerprint check for all nurses applying for licensure by endorsement, some will require proof of current competency as a nurse, and some will require that you take a particular course before, or soon after, being licensed in the state.

Temporary Permit

Most states issue a temporary permit that allows the endorsement applicant to practice in the state for a limited period of time while the remaining requirements are met. This can be useful if you plan to move to that state immediately and would like to begin work soon. There is an additional fee for a temporary permit.

Nurse Licensure Compact

The Nurse Licensure Compact is an agreement between a number of U.S. states that allows nurses who permanently reside in, and are licensed in, one of these states to practice in all of them. As of 2008, there are 23 states participating in the Nurse Licensure Compact.

The Compact includes language regarding recognition of licensure, discipline, information sharing, and other provisions. If a nurse is a permanent resident of a state that is in the Compact, then that state is considered the nurse's "home" state. That state's Board of Nursing issues the nursing license. This license then grants the nurse the privilege to practice in other states (called "party states") that are members of the Compact.

Location of Nursing Practice

The Compact defines nursing practice as occurring where the patient is located; thus, a nurse is required to follow the regulations of the Compact state in which he or she is practicing. If you move out of a Compact state and become a resident of a state that is not in the Compact, you no longer have a multistate license. At that point, your license converts to a single-state license and is only valid in the state that issued it.

Nurse Licensure Compact States
◆ - Compact States
◉ - Non Compact States

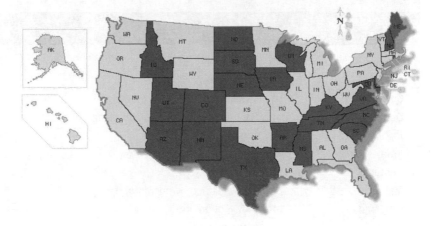

Figure 4.1. Nurse licensure compact states, 2008.

Mutual recognition of a nurse's license in states belonging to the Compact increases nurse mobility and facilitates delivery of health care by innovative communication practices, such as **telenursing.** Figure 4.1 illustrates the 23 Compact states on a map of the United States.

Table 4.3 lists those states that have implemented the Nurse Licensure Compact and their Web addresses as of the end of 2008.

Seeking a license in the United States can be costly, involving fees for immigration, licensure applications, transcripts, credentials evaluation, and others. To prepare you for these costs, and to assist you in keeping track of what you have paid, a form is included in Appendix C.

THE ROLE OF CGFNS INTERNATIONAL

CGFNS International (formerly known as the Commission on Graduates of Foreign Nursing Schools) protects the public by ensuring

Table 4.3

LIST OF STATES IN THE NURSE LICENSURE COMPACT AND WEB ADDRESSES

STATE BOARD OF NURSING	WEB ADDRESS
Arizona	http://www.azbn.gov/
Arkansas	http://www.arsbn.org/
Colorado	http://www.dora.state.co.us/nursing/
Delaware	http://dpr.delaware.gov/boards/nursing/
Idaho	http://www2.state.id.us/ibn
Iowa	http://www.iowa.gov/nursing
Kentucky	http://www.kbn.ky.gov/
Maine	http://www.maine.gov/boardofnursing/
Maryland	http://www.mbon.org/
Mississippi	http://www.msbn.state.ms.us/
Nebraska	http://www.hhs.state.ne.us/crl/nursing/nursingindex.htm
New Hampshire	http://www.state.nh.us/nursing/
New Mexico	http://www.bon.state.nm.us/
North Carolina	http://www.ncbon.com/
North Dakota	http://www.ndbon.org/
Rhode Island	http://www.health.ri.gov/
South Carolina	http://www.llr.state.sc.us/pol/nursing
South Dakota	http://www.state.sd.us/doh/nursing/
Tennessee	http://health.state.tn.us/Boards/Nursing/index.htm
Texas	http://www.bon.state.tx.us
Utah	http://www.dopl.utah.gov/licensing/nursing.html
Virginia	http://www.dhp.virginia.gov/nursing/
Wisconsin	http://drl.wi.gov/

that nurses and other health care professionals educated outside the United States are eligible and qualified to meet licensure, immigration, and other U.S. practice requirements. Most states require a foreign-educated nurse who is seeking U.S. licensure to complete one or more of the following CGFNS programs.

CGFNS Certification Program (CP)

The CGFNS Certification Program (CP) is designed specifically for first-level, generalist (registered or professional) nurses educated outside the United States who are eligible to practice as RNs in the United States. The program consists of three parts:

- *A credentials review,* which includes an evaluation of secondary and nursing education, registration, and licensure. To be eligible for the CGFNS Qualifying Exam^{SM}, you must have completed a sufficient number of hours of classroom instruction and clinical practice in adult health (medical/surgical) nursing, maternal/infant nursing, nursing of children, and psychiatric/ mental health nursing. If you have not completed a sufficient number of hours in each of these areas, you will not be eligible to take the CGFNS Qualifying Exam until you complete an entire course (both theory and clinical) in the deficient area(s) at a government-approved nursing school in the United States or elsewhere.
- *The CGFNS Qualifying Exam,* which is a test of nursing knowledge that is offered up to four times a year in over 55 test sites worldwide. Each exam is given on the same day all over the world and takes an entire day. Each time the CGFNS examination is given, new test questions are used. This examination tests your basic level of knowledge in nursing. To be eligible to take the CGFNS Qualifying Exam, you must have graduated from a government-approved first-level, general (RN) nursing program that included at least 2 years of general nursing education, and you must hold initial and current licensure as a general nurse in your country of education. Persons licensed solely as midwives, pediatric nurses, psychiatric nurses, or other specialty nurses (i.e., without also being educated and licensed to practice general nursing) are not eligible for the CGFNS Qualifying Exam. Successful completion of this examination also satisfies one of the immigration requirements for securing an occupational visa to work in the United States. For a listing

of CGFNS examination centers and test dates, please see the CGFNS Web site at http://www.cgfns.org/sections/programs/cp/cp-qe.shtml.

■ *An English language proficiency examination* unless you are exempt from English language testing. You may take either TOEFL (Test of English as a Foreign Language: required score = 207), TOEFL iBT (Internet-based TOEFL: required score = 83), TOEIC (Test of English for International Communication: required score = 725), or IELTS (International English Language Testing System: required score = 6.5 Overall in the Academic module) to complete this requirement. You must contact the English language test provider directly to apply for English language testing. The score report (results of the English testing) must be sent directly to CGFNS by the test provider and to the Board of Nursing if the Board requires the report. Information on how to contact the testing organizations may be found in the CGFNS Certification Program Handbook or online at http://www.cgfns.org/sections/programs/cp/cp-english.shtml.

English Language Exemptions

To be exempt from English language testing, you must meet the following criteria: your nursing education program must have been in English using English textbooks and must have been located in Australia, Barbados, Canada (except Quebec—only students who graduated from McGill University or Dawson University in Montreal, Vanier College in Saint Laurent, John Abbot College in Sainte-Anne-de-Bellevue, or Heritage College in Gatineau are exempt from the English language requirement of the Certification Program), Ireland, Jamaica, New Zealand, South Africa, Trinidad and Tobago, or the United Kingdom.

Upon successful completion of the Certification Program, you will be issued a CP certificate. This certificate is required of foreign-educated RNs by many U.S. states if they are to take the U.S. licensure examination, the NCLEX-RN.

CGFNS Credentials Evaluation Service (CES)

The CGFNS Credentials Evaluation Service (CES) analyzes the credentials of RNs and LPN/LVNs who were educated outside of the United States and who wish to pursue licensure or academic admission in the United States. The CES provides a report that is advisory in nature and does not make specific placement recommendations. The analysis and reporting process generally takes from 6 to 8 weeks after receipt of all required documentation and fees. Processing times may vary during periods of high volume. Once completed, the CES report is submitted to the Board of Nursing, school, employer, or other entity, and a copy is sent to you.

The resulting CES report serves as a valuable tool for regulatory and licensing agencies and helps to demonstrate the merits of your credentials compared to U.S. standards. There are two types of CES reports: a full education course-by-course report and a Health Care Profession and Science Report. You should contact the Board of Nursing that has requested the report to find out which type of report they require. A copy of each type of report is included in Appendix D.

CGFNS/ICHP VisaScreen Program

A number of State Boards of Nursing will accept your VisaScreen certificate as meeting the credentials evaluation for licensure in that state. The VisaScreen program requires that your education be deemed comparable to that of a nurse educated in the United States; that all licenses held by you are determined to be valid and unencumbered; that you have demonstrated the required proficiency in written and oral English; and, for RNs, that you have passed a test of nursing knowledge—either the CGFNS Qualifying Exam or the NCLEX-RN examination (see chapter 3 for an in-depth discussion of the VisaScreen program and its requirements). You should contact the State Board of Nursing in your intended state of practice to determine if they accept the VisaScreen certificate for licensure purposes.

CGFNS New York Credentials Verification Service

The New York Credentials Verification Service for New York State independently collects and verifies the authenticity of your education, licensure, and registration credentials. Requests for education and licensure validation must be submitted to your school and licensing authority by CGFNS, which also will pay the appropriate fees. Once verified, the documents are forwarded to the New York State Education Department (NYSED) to be evaluated as part of your licensure application. Only applicants applying for licensure in New York are required to complete the New York Credentials Verification Service. If you hold a CP certificate, NYSED may grant a limited permit to practice for a year without requiring passage of the NCLEX-RN examination. You would be required to practice under the supervision of an RN until you passed the NCLEX examination and obtained your state license.

Documents Required for CGFNS Programs

In order for CGFNS to complete an evaluation of your credentials for the CP, CES, or VisaScreen programs, the following documents are required. Applications may be submitted online, but all documentation must be sent to CGFNS by mail.

- A completed application form and full payment for the program/service to which you are applying.
- A full transcript (and, in the case of the CP program, a completed Nursing Education Form) with an official school seal/stamp, mailed directly to CGFNS from your school, verifying the total number of hours of classroom instruction (theory) and hours/days of clinical practice you completed in each of the nursing courses your took during your education program.
- A validation of your original and current registration/licensure as a first-level, generalist nurse (RN), mailed to CGFNS directly from the authority that issues registrations/licensure in your original country of education (CP program only).

- A validation of your initial license and all subsequent licenses as an RN or LPN/LVN, mailed to CGFNS directly by the licensing authority that issued the licenses (CES requires validation of initial licensure and all other non-U.S. licenses and VisaScreen requires validation of all licenses U.S. and non-U.S. issued).
- A copy of your secondary school diploma. If you no longer have your original diploma, an official letter with the school seal/stamp and signed by the principal may be sent to CGFNS directly from your secondary school, verifying your dates of attendance and date of completion/graduation.

Transcripts

Some applicants find that there is no longer an official record from their nursing education program. Perhaps the school has been closed and the records destroyed—or perhaps the political situation in the country prevents access to any remaining records. In that case, CGFNS will accept copies of documents from you or other regulatory bodies for comparison with its historical database on nursing education worldwide.

Such cases are reviewed by the CGFNS Professional Nurse Credentials and Standards Committee or the Licensed Practical Nurse Standards Committee for a final decision. The Standards Committees are composed of members of the profession (generally educators and regulatory personnel), an admissions officer from a college or university, and a public member.

If you have previously had transcripts sent to CGFNS for one of its programs, CGFNS can produce certified copies of nursing education records upon your request. Many licensure boards and academic organizations will accept educational documents from CGFNS in cases where they cannot be obtained from the school.

The CGFNS Qualifying Exam

The CGFNS Qualifying Exam is a paper and pencil test that evaluates the nursing knowledge of foreign-educated, first level, general nurses

(RNs). It consists of 265 questions, with 150 questions being administered in the A.M. testing session and 115 questions administered in the P.M. testing session. The CGFNS Qualifying Exam was originally designed to predict success on the U.S. licensure examination for RNs, and thus, it uses the same test blueprint as the NCLEX-RN examination.

Test Blueprint

The test blueprint, or test plan, is divided into four major client (patient) need categories. The content of each category is related to the level of nursing knowledge of a U.S. nurse within 6 months of entry into practice. In other words, each content area tests what a nurse practicing in the United States should know 6 months into his or her nursing career. The four major client need categories are: safe effective care environment, health promotion and maintenance, psychosocial integrity, and physiological integrity (NCSBN, 2007).

Safe, effective care environment: This category focuses on achieving client outcomes by providing and directing nursing care in such a way as to protect clients, family/significant others, and other health care personnel. Subcategories include management of care and safety and infection control.

Health promotion and maintenance: This category focuses on providing and directing nursing care across the life span. That care is based on knowledge of expected growth and development principles, prevention or early detection of health problems, and strategies to achieve optimal health.

Psychosocial integrity: This category focuses on providing and directing nursing care that promotes and supports the emotional, mental, and social well-being of the client and family/significant others experiencing stressful events, as well as clients with acute or chronic mental illness.

Physiological integrity: This category focuses on providing and directing nursing care that promotes physical health and wellness by: (1) providing comfort and assistance related to client performance of activities of daily living; (2) providing care related to the administration of medications and parenteral therapies; (3) providing care that reduces the likelihood that clients will develop complications or health problems related to existing conditions, treatments, or procedures; and (4) managing and providing care to clients with acute, chronic, or life-threatening physical health conditions.

Exam Question Format

The CGFNS Qualifying Exam uses objective, multiple-choice questions. With this type of format you are given the question and four possible answers, only one of which is correct. You are required to choose the best answer to the question.

In 2004, CGFNS introduced several different types of questions into its examination. These are called alternate item types and include such things as charts, graphs, and multiple correct answer and short answer questions. These types of questions were introduced because of their use on the NCLEX-RN examination. You may see one or two of these types of questions on the CGFNS Qualifying Exam that you take.

Diagnostic Profile and Score Report

Examination results are posted to the CGFNS Web site 4 weeks following the test date. Your results letter is included in the posting and contains your pass/fail status, your score on the examination, and a **diagnostic profile.**

The diagnostic profile gives you a graphic representation of how well you performed in each client need category on the examination. You may access your score results by logging onto the CGFNS Web site at http://www.cgfns.org and clicking on CGFNS Connect-Apply/Check Status. Then click on Login-Check Your Status, and it will take you to a password protected part of the CGFNS Web site. You will have to enter your login and password to access your test results. A copy of a *Pass* letter with a diagnostic profile, a *Fail* letter with a diagnostic profile, and an explanation of the client need categories is included in Appendix D.

CGFNS Preparation for the Licensure Examination

CGFNS provides opportunities for you to assess your readiness for the NCLEX-RN examination before beginning the licensure application process. One way to predict your readiness for the NCLEX-RN examination is through the CGFNS Certification Program and its Qualifying Exam, offered up to four times a year in numerous locations around the world. Since the introduction of the certification program, first-time RN-licensure pass rates of foreign-educated nurses holding a CGFNS certificate has increased from about 15% to 20% (prior to the Certification Program in the 1970s) to 85% to 90% (CGFNS, 2007).

Another resource to prepare for both the CGFNS Qualifying Exam and the licensure examination is through the Kaplan/CGFNS Advantage Program, Knowledge for Nursing. This program provides educational materials online and offline to provide nurses with what they need to prepare for and pass the examinations. You may access information on this program at http://www.kaplancgfns.com.

THE NCLEX EXAMINATIONS

The NCLEX examinations are developed by the National Council of State Boards of Nursing, Inc. (NCSBN). NCSBN originally was "organized to provide a forum where its member Boards could meet together to discuss matters of common interest and concern that impact the health, safety, and welfare of the public." NCSBN's current mission is that "the National Council of State Boards of Nursing, composed of member boards, provides leadership to advance regulatory excellence for public protection" (NCSBN, 2008b).

NCSBN is made up of Boards of Nursing from all 50 states, the District of Columbia, and four U.S. territories—American Samoa, Guam, Northern Mariana Islands, and the Virgin Islands. It also has an associate member category designed for international nursing regulatory bodies, and it considers membership in that category at its annual meeting. The member Boards act together to ensure that safe and competent nursing care is provided by all licensed nurses.

Development of the NCLEX Examinations

Practice Analysis

The content of the items on the NCLEX examinations is based on a practice analysis of entry-level nurses working in the United States and is conducted every 3 years. This means that newly licensed nurses practicing in the United States are surveyed to collect data on the current practice of the entry-level nurse. Findings from the practice analysis help NCSBN to evaluate the NCLEX test plans that guide the content of the licensure examinations. The NCLEX-RN and NCLEX-PN test plans for candidates are available at the NCSBN Web site (http://www.ncsbn.org/1287.htm) and will provide helpful information and guidance as you prepare for the examination.

As you prepare for the licensure examination, keep in mind that it is about basic, entry-level nursing interventions. All items are developed and validated using the expertise of practicing nurses, educators, and nursing regulators from throughout the United States.

NCLEX Statistics

In 2008, the pass rate for foreign-educated nurses who took the NCLEX-RN examination was 36.8%, compared to 80% for U.S.-educated RN candidates. For those foreign-educated nurses who took the NCLEX-PN examination during 2008, the pass rate was 33.6% compared to 77.9% for U.S.-educated LPN/LVN candidates.

The top five countries of origin for foreign-educated nurses who took either the NCLEX-RN or NCLEX-PN examination for the first time in 2008 were the Philippines, India, South Korea, Cuba, and Canada (NCSBN, 2008c).

Applying for the NCLEX

To take the NCLEX examination, you will first need to apply for licensure by examination to a Board of Nursing, and you should contact the individual Board of Nursing for the process and requirements of the state in which you intend to practice. The licensure process can begin before you are actually in the United States. Obtaining a license requires strict adherence to the requirements of the state or territory in which you are seeking licensure. Therefore, pay particular attention to the application instructions.

Keeping Records

You should keep a copy of all documents and communications for future reference. Do not assume that the Board of Nursing or other organization will be able to locate your records. By keeping copies of your documents, you can help the Board or any other organization track the documents if your records are misplaced, misfiled, or have never even arrived.

A tracking form is included in Appendix C to help you keep up with what was sent, where it was sent, and when you either mailed it or asked that it be mailed. You can also make notes regarding when you spoke to someone from the Board about your application.

Special Accommodations

If you will require special testing accommodations because of special needs (such as those related to a disability), you will need to obtain permission from the Board of Nursing. Each Board has instructions on how to apply for such accommodations and what kind of medical or other documentation is required.

Register and Pay for the NCLEX Examination With Pearson VUE

NCSBN contracts with a test service company, Pearson VUE, for development and administration of the NCLEX examinations. You will need to contact Pearson VUE when you begin the application process for the NCLEX examination, and you can do so online, by phone, or by mail. When completing the registration form, enter your name exactly as it is printed on the identification that you will present at the test center when you take the examination.

You must pay for the NCLEX examination by credit card if registering online or by telephone. If registering by mail you may pay by credit card, a certified check, a cashier's check, or a money order in U.S. currency and drawn on a U.S. bank. Personal checks are not accepted under any circumstances, and no refunds are issued for any reason.

Receive Eligibility From Your Board of Nursing

Once both your state licensure application and your NCLEX application have been received, the Board of Nursing will determine if you are eligible for licensure by examination in that state. If it determines that you are eligible, the Board will then notify Pearson VUE that you are eligible to test.

Receive Authorization to Test

Once Pearson VUE receives notification from the Board of Nursing that you are eligible to test, they will send you an Authorization to Test (ATT). You must have your ATT in order to schedule a testing appointment.

Keep this document in a secure place because you will need to present it at the testing center on the day of your examination, and you will not be admitted without it. The name on this ATT must match exactly the name you entered when you registered for the examination and the identification that you will bring with you to the test center for admission. If the names do not match exactly, you may be denied admission to the test center.

Schedule Your Examination

You must take the examination within the test dates listed on your ATT. These dates are determined by the Board of Nursing and cannot be extended for any reason. It is recommended that you make your appointment to test as soon as possible after receiving your ATT, even though you might not be testing immediately. This will give you the greatest number of options in selecting the date and time that is best for you.

If you would like to take your examination at a center outside of the United States, you must contact customer service at Pearson VUE directly. All test sessions outside of the United States require an additional international scheduling fee plus a value-added tax where applicable.

The Examination Experience

Checking In at the Testing Center

You should plan to arrive at the testing center about 30 minutes before your scheduled appointment. If the center is in an area with which you are not familiar, you should locate it before the day of the examination. If you arrive more than 30 minutes late for your scheduled appointment, then you may not be allowed to take the test—you may be required to forfeit your registration fee and to re-register and pay a new registration fee in order to test at a later date. The Board of Nursing would then have to issue another ATT before you can schedule another testing appointment.

When you arrive at the testing center, you will be required to show your ATT and proof of identification. You will be photographed, and you will have a digital fingerprint taken before you are taken into the testing room. There are three acceptable forms of identification for test centers located in the United States—a passport, an identification card issued by a U.S. state or territory, or a driver's license issued by a U.S. state or territory. If you are testing in a center outside of the United States, the only acceptable form of identification is a passport. All forms of identification must be valid, must be current, must be in English, must contain a photograph and signature, and must be signed in English.

The Testing Session

The NCLEX examinations are given in computer format. However, it is not necessary for you to know how to use a computer before you take the examination. Your session will begin with a tutorial to familiarize you with the types of items on the examination, how to proceed through the examination, how to use the keys on the computer, how to record your answer, how to use the on-screen calculator, and other related points.

Once you have completed the tutorial, the examination will begin and will continue until it has been determined that you are either above or below the passing standard. All testing sessions are monitored by proctors as well as by video and audio recordings.

The Examination

You will have up to 6 hours to complete the NCLEX-RN examination and up to 5 hours to complete the NCLEX-PN examination. This includes the tutorial, the testing time, and all breaks.

There are a minimum of 75 questions and a maximum of 265 questions on the NCLEX-RN examination and a minimum of 85 questions and a maximum of 205 questions on the NCLEX-PN examination. It is not possible to predict how many questions your examination will have because the computer selects questions for each candidate as he or she takes the examination—each question is based on your response to the previous question.

Computer Adaptive Testing

The NCLEX examinations are computer adaptive. This means that every time you answer a question, the computer recalculates your ability and selects the next item that is the best match to that ability level. Testing stops when it can be determined with 95% confidence that your performance is either above or below the passing standard, regardless of the number of items you answered or the amount of testing time elapsed. Testing also will stop when the maximum amount of time has passed or when the maximum number of questions has been answered. It is a good idea to pace yourself as you move through the test.

Question Types

The examination is primarily made up of multiple-choice questions that have one best answer. However, there are some other types of questions on the examination, including multiple response items (items with one or more correct answers that require you to select all of the correct answers), items that require you to make a mathematical calculation and then fill in the blank with the answer, and items that require you to reorder the options to be in the correct order. You can view the different item types in the tutorial provided on the NCSBN and Pearson VUE Web sites for candidates.

Results

No results are provided to you at the testing center, nor are any results provided to you from Pearson VUE or from NCSBN. Only Boards of Nursing can release NCLEX examination results to candidates. Some Boards of Nursing participate in the NCSBN Quick Results Service, which means that, if you pay a fee, you can receive unofficial results by phone within a few days after the examination. Official results are received directly from the Board of Nursing within a few weeks of the examination.

Repeating the Examination

If you do not pass the examination, you will receive a **diagnostic report** that summarizes your strengths and weaknesses. This report can be used to guide you as you prepare to retake the examination. You will need to reapply with a Board of Nursing and with Pearson VUE as a repeat candidate.

Most states allow you to retest after 45 days, although some have a longer waiting period. Each state sets its own policies regarding how many times a candidate may take the examination. If you are taking the examination as a repeat candidate, you will not receive any test items that you have seen within the past year (NCSBN, 2008a).

SUMMARY

Obtaining a license to practice as a nurse in the United States can be a lengthy and complicated process for foreign-educated nurses. Using this chapter as a guide, you should be able to work through the steps and assemble the documents you need. It is important to remember that each Board of Nursing is responsible for licensure within that state or territory and that differences do exist among the states. Therefore, regularly check the Web site of the Board in which you are interested and take note of changes and announcements within that state that might impact your licensure.

RESOURCES

- For NCLEX candidate information, including a list of test centers, a tutorial, and other NCLEX information, see: http://www.pearsonvue.com/nclex.
- For a list of State Boards of Nursing contact information and the Nurse Licensure Compact, see: http://www.ncsbn.org.
- For information on the CGFNS Certification Program, Credentials Evaluation Service, VisaScreen program, and New York Verification Service, including instructions, applications, and other information, see: http://www.cgfns.org.
- For information on the NCLEX-RN and NCLEX-PN examinations, including instructions, application, and additional information, see: http://www.ncsbn.org.
- For Kaplan/CGFNS Advantage, Knowledge for Nursing (preparation for the NCLEX and CGFNS examinations), see: http://www.kaplancgfns.com.
- For English language proficiency examination information, see: http://www.ets.org, http://www.toefl.org, http://www.ets.org/tse, or http://www.ets.org/toeic for TOEFL, TWE, TSE, or TOEIC; see: http://www.ielts.org for the IELTS examination.
- For U.S. immigration services and benefits and for visa information, see: http://www.uscis.gov/portal/site/uscis.

REFERENCES

Commission on Graduates of Foreign Nursing Schools. (2007). *CGFNS validity study 2006–2007*. Philadelphia, PA: Author.
National Council of State Boards of Nursing. (2007). *NCSBN member board profiles*. Chicago, IL: Author.

National Council of State Boards of Nursing. (2008a). *NCLEX examination candidate bulletin*. Chicago, IL: Author. Retrieved January 29, 2009, from: http://www.ncsbn.org/2008_NCLEX_Candidate_Bulletin.pdf

National Council of State Boards of Nursing. (2008b). *NCSBN fact sheet: Organizational overview: 2008*. Retrieved January 28, 2009, from: http://www.ncsbn.org/NCSBN_Fact_Sheet_December__2008.pdf

National Council of State Boards of Nursing. (2008c). *NCSBN quarterly examination statistics: Volume, pass rates and first-time internationally educated candidates' countries in 2008*. Retrieved January 29, 2009, from: http://www.ncsbn.org/NCLEX_Stats_2008_Q4.pdf

U.S. Bill of Rights (n.d.). Retrieved January 28, 2009, from: http://www.archives.gov/exhibits/charters/bill_of_rights_transcript.html

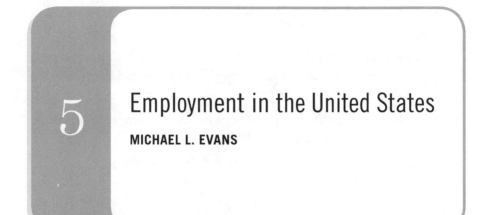

5 Employment in the United States

MICHAEL L. EVANS

In This Chapter

Keywords

Collective bargaining: Negotiations between management and a union about pay and conditions of employment on behalf of all the workers in the union.

Congruence: Internal and external consistency; conformity or agreement.

Cultural competence: An ability to interact effectively with people of different cultures.

Extended care facilities: Medical institutions that provide prolonged care (as in cases of prolonged illness or rehabilitation from acute illness).

Mandatory overtime: Where employers *require* employees to work more than the standard 40 hours per week.

Professional autonomy: Responsible discretionary decision making by a profession or an individual within the profession; the quality or condition of being self-governing.

Shared governance: A set of practices under which management and staff join in decision making.

Video conference: Live audio and visual transmission of meeting activities to bring people at different sites together.

Voluntary overtime: Where an employee offers or agrees to work for pay in excess of the standard 40 hours per week.

The previous chapters have described the various visa and licensing requirements necessary for foreign-educated nurses to practice nursing in the United States. This chapter provides information on the characteristics of a supportive work environment and reviews employee rights and obligations. While you may have selected a geographical area of the country in which to live based on personal preferences—such as the presence of family or friends, the climate, or the cost of living—there are still many important factors to consider when selecting a workplace. We hope you find this chapter helpful in finding and obtaining employment in an organization that meets your expectations and gives you a long, fulfilling career.

SELECTING A WORKPLACE

Choosing the Right Practice Setting

As discussed in previous chapters, nurses working in the United States have a variety of practice settings to choose from when planning a career, including hospitals that care for acutely ill patients, long-term care facilities such as nursing homes, and agencies that provide care for homebound patients in the community, to name a few. Use your previous nursing experience as a guide to evaluating which type of practice setting is best for your first job in the United States. While you may wish to start working in a new nursing specialty or a different type of facility immediately upon entry, keep in mind that your transition to working and living in the United States may be a stressful time and that you may face many challenges in your personal and professional life.

The majority of nurses in the United States work in hospitals. According to the 2004 National Sample Survey of Registered Nurses conducted by the Bureau of Health Professions, 59.1% of U.S. nurses worked in hospitals, 18.2% in public health or community health settings, 9.5% in ambulatory care settings, and 6.9% in nursing homes and **extended care facilities.** However, the fastest growing segments of nursing employment continue to be in ambulatory care, followed by public and community health (Bureau of Health Professions, 2004). Figure 5.1 presents the percent change in the number of registered nurses (RNs) employed in selected U.S. health care settings from 1980 to 2004.

What to Look For in a Workplace

No matter what type of practice setting you choose, you will want to work in a facility that provides a supportive environment for its nurses, including its foreign-educated nurses. Check with your prospective employer to see what resources are available to nurses new to the United States and if there is an acculturation program available for foreign-educated nurses. If there is not such a program, ask if you can speak to a current employee who was educated abroad so that you can learn from his/her experiences. Pay particular attention to the orientation programs available, the health care management style and philosophy, and the climate of the workplace environment.

Orientation Program

Orientation is a period of time during which you will learn about the hospital, your unit, and the skills and competencies required for

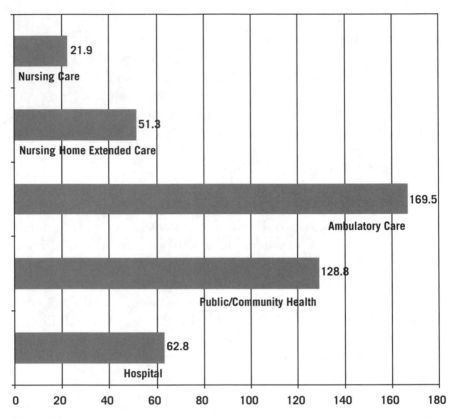

Figure 5.1. Percent change in the number of registered nurses employed in selected U.S. health care settings from 1980 to 2004.
Source: The Registered Nurse Population: Findings from the 2004 National Sample Survey of Registered Nurses, Bureau of Health Professions, Health Resources and Services Administration.

performing well in your job. Orientation programs differ in terms of length of time, how structured they are, and what kinds of experiences they provide.

Orientations can range from 4 weeks to 6 months, sometimes longer, but all are designed to assist with your transition to nursing in your new place of employment. Orientation is often divided into two phases: (1) overall orientation to the facility, and (2) orientation to the specific unit on which you will work.

Content

Orientation to the facility may include such things as review of general policies and procedures, structure of the facility, organizational charts that show how each unit functions in a facility, a description of the health care system, and the role of nursing within the institution. Orientation to the facility also may include a test of your knowledge of medications, medication administration, and simple math. It may be administered during the general orientation or prior to beginning work on your assigned unit.

More specific orientations will include an introduction to the unit and staff, and to unit functions, such as work schedules, patient assignments, shift reports and handling emergency situations. More specific orientations also may include new methods of administering medication and other uses of technology in providing care.

Hospitals report that within the varied lengths of orientation they are providing English classes and classes in medical terminology, which include slang terms, idioms, and abbreviations commonly used in U.S. nursing practice to benefit foreign-educated nurses. Other modifications of orientation include conducting classes in **cultural competence,** developing informal social networks, facilitating housing, providing a "buddy" system, and creating a mentor or preceptor system (Davis, 2005).

You may want to ask questions about how long the orientation program will be, if it includes classes or other formal learning experiences, and if you will be assigned to work with a preceptor. A preceptor is an experienced nurse who will help you to become fully acquainted with the workplace, the health care institution's policies and procedures, and your role as a professional nurse in that institution and unit.

Most important is to recognize that anxiety almost always accompanies new experiences. Such anxiety is sometimes unavoidable, but it can be minimized by taking the following steps prior to your scheduled orientation:

- *Know what is expected of you:* Should you wear a uniform, or can you wear regular dress clothes on your first day of orientation? Find out what documents you will need to have with you (e.g. nursing license, social security card, health records, etc.). Each facility is different, so know what is required before you arrive. You should receive a letter of hire from the employing institution directly or from your recruiter or immigration attorney (if you have used either).

■ *Know how to get there:* What time should you be at the facility and in what room/location? Take a trial run by practicing the route you will take, and know how long it will take if you are walking, driving, or taking public transportation. Allow extra time for emergencies or disruptions in transportation. Plan on arriving at least 10–15 minutes early.

Educational Resources

Additionally, you should ask about educational resources that are available to employees. Many health care employers offer tuition reimbursement, through which employers will pay all or some of nurses' tuition expenses if they return to school to continue their education.

Not all employers offer tuition reimbursement. Among those that do, the amount of reimbursement and other factors—such as whether courses need to be taken at specific schools, whether they must be in nursing (or whether they may be in another field), and whether reimbursement is available only after a nurse has worked for the employer for a specific amount of time—will vary considerably between hospitals.

Some employers also will pay some of the costs of brief continuing education courses. Some will provide workplace-based continuing education in your specialty area that can help you to stay abreast of new developments and increase the level of your professional performance.

Management Style and Philosophy

The management style and philosophy of a facility and unit are also important aspects to consider when seeking employment. Many hospitals employ a **shared governance** model, in which nurses are directly involved in decision-making processes about matters that affect the workplace. An example of shared governance is the use of a professional practice council, in which nurses from each unit or department are selected by their coworkers to participate in a committee that makes recommendations to nursing administration about nursing practice and workplace issues.

Workplace Environment

Another factor to consider is the unit climate, sometimes called the workplace environment, which includes the level of job satisfaction among staff nurses and the quality of interpersonal interaction among staff nurses, management, and other professionals in a clinical area. Some of the factors that influence unit climate include how well staff relate to and communicate with each other and how well they perform as a team. Each of these factors contributes to creating a supportive work environment for staff nurses, which in turn can improve nurses' job satisfaction and the quality of patient care.

What Are Magnet Hospitals?

In the mid-1990s, the American Nurses Association (ANA), through the American Nurses Credentialing Center (ANCC), created the Magnet Recognition Program. This program certifies hospitals that empower nurses, through education and managerial support, to provide high-quality patient care and that support **professional autonomy** and development (Kramer & Schmalenberg, 2004).

Magnet certification has become the gold standard for professional nursing practice. Magnet hospitals have been found to attract and retain nurses at higher rates than non-Magnet hospitals, support the provision of high-quality nursing care, and achieve high levels of nurse job satisfaction. A complete listing of Magnet facilities is available at the following Web site: http://www.nursecredentialing.org/MagnetOrg/searchmagnet.cfm.

Getting Information About Employment Opportunities

Recruitment agencies are often good sources for learning of specific job openings. Local newspapers (often available online) and some Web-based resources (such as http://www.monster.com and http://www.healthecareers.com) are also sources of information on current job openings. Many U.S. health care institutions maintain Web sites that provide information on the institution, including open positions.

Web sites frequently give valuable information about employment qualifications, benefits, and the type and length of orientation programs provided for new nurses. Many employers now offer the option of applying for positions online.

OBTAINING A JOB

After you have decided where you would like to live, the type of facility in which you would like to work, and the workplace characteristics and benefits that are important to you, it is time to concentrate on getting the job. By now, you should have prepared your résumé and/or portfolio (see chapter 2, "Developing Your Portfolio") and are ready to apply for a job either through a recruiter, a facility that has recruited you, or on your own. If you have not developed your résumé or would like to update it, consider the following guidelines for constructing a résumé and a cover letter for prospective employers.

Preparing a Résumé

A résumé is a document that summarizes your employment history and educational background. Employers usually require applicants to submit a résumé in addition to completing an application form. Many also require a cover letter that highlights the relevant aspects of your professional experience and explains your interest in, and qualifications for, the announced position.

Your résumé is an employer's first introduction to you, and it is important that you take the time to write it well. It will give the employer an idea of who you are professionally and what your career goals are. The résumé can be submitted on paper by regular mail, and often it can be submitted online through the employer's Web site or by e-mail. Check to see if a potential employer prefers or requires a specific means of submitting your résumé.

Personal Information

Résumés follow a similar general format and require specific information about you, including: your full legal name, mailing address, telephone number, and e-mail address; your professional objective (reason for applying for the position), educational institutions attended, and degrees earned; professional experience; licensure; professional organization affiliation; honors and awards received; and references.

Your résumé should never include identifying information such as your work authorization number, visa or social security number, or personal information such as your marital status, number of children, or a photograph of yourself. Be sure to write the résumé in the third person, avoiding "I" or "me" statements. Keep the information concise, limiting yourself to one or two pages.

Professional Objective

A statement of your professional objective should describe short-term and long-term professional goals. You should review the information available about the employer so that you have a good idea of what positions are open and match your qualifications.

An example of your short-term goal might be to list the clinical areas for which you are qualified and that you would like to be employed in one of those areas. An example of your long-term goal would be what you ultimately hope to achieve in nursing, such as a position in administration or quality assurance or higher degrees you hope to achieve.

Education

Education should be outlined in reverse chronological order—that is, it should start with the most recent (or current) education and continue back through secondary school. You should include all degrees you have earned, naming the institutions you attended, their location, your program of study, and dates of attendance. This section of the résumé also includes any certifications or special training, where you received them, and the date you completed them.

Professional Experience

The section on professional experience should be easy to read and should answer the question, "What do you know how to do?" This information should also be listed in reverse chronological order. You should first list your current or previous employer, location, position held, dates employed, and a brief description of your responsibilities. This is where you should showcase special skills you have obtained as a result of positions you have held. Your résumé should list all positions you have held, even those that were outside of nursing and health care.

Licensure

The licensure section should answer the questions, "What job can you do, and where can you do it?" If you are already licensed in the United States, you should include the specific state(s) in which you are licensed to practice. If you are already licensed in the state in which you plan to work, or if your licensure is pending, you should be sure to include this fact. Additionally, you should list any professional organizations to which you belong and any honors or awards you have received in the past.

References

In the final section, References, you may simply state that "References will be provided upon request." Or, you may list your references, in which case you should generally include three references, at least two of them from people with whom you have worked. Some employers may specify that they want you to include references when you submit your résumé.

When listing professional references be sure to include the person's full credentials, such as "Susan Smith, PhD, RN," and title, as well as current address, telephone numbers, and e-mail address for each reference you list. Be sure to contact your references to ask for permission to use their names before you submit your résumé. You can find examples of résumés and résumé formats online at various sites, including http://resume.monster.com, and a sample in Appendix A.

Preparing a Cover Letter

When sending your résumé to a potential employer, you always should include a cover letter. Your letter should explain why you are applying for this particular position and why you believe that you are a good match for it. If possible, you also should indicate something about what you know of the organization and how you will fit in with the workplace culture. At the end of the cover letter, you should indicate that you anticipate and look forward to being interviewed. You should not inquire about salary or benefits in your cover letter, as those discussions will occur later in the interview process.

When preparing your résumé and cover letter, consider asking someone you trust to proofread them for typographical, spelling, or grammatical errors. Finally, make sure your résumé and cover letter are neat and visually appealing. Using a high-quality, lightly colored paper, such as a soft gray, may help your résumé stand out. A sample cover letter is provided in Appendix A.

Recruitment Agencies

There are many agencies that seek to recruit around the world for jobs in the United States. Many of these recruitment agencies can assess a foreign-educated nurse's chances of being successful in finding a job and should be able to assist with preparing for the NCLEX examination. They also may be able to assess the nurse's English language proficiency, educational preparation, and career experience.

Nurses outside of the United States should seek recruiters who can help them to manage possible social and cultural isolation after moving to another country. Some international nursing recruitment agencies offer acculturation programs for nurses who move to the United States in order to help them adjust successfully.

Staffing Agencies

In the United States, many staffing agencies supply nurses for temporary or short-term assignments in health care facilities. Typically, the employer pays the staffing agency, which then pays the nurse. Working through a staffing agency often provides nurses with greater variety and flexibility than working directly for a hospital or other facility, especially in regard to scheduling. However, it also provides less stability—for example, an assignment may be canceled with little notice.

Most staffing agencies focus on providing temporary staffing in a specific, geographical area (e.g., a metropolitan area). On the other hand, some staffing agencies focus on providing "traveling nurses" for temporary assignments that may be in a distant state. Many nurses find working through a "traveling" agency desirable, at least for a little while, because it offers opportunities for travel around the country. Such assignments are usually for a period that lasts from several weeks to several months. For more in-depth information on recruitment and staffing agencies, see chapter 2.

Interviewing

As a nurse looking for a job in the United States, your interview might be arranged by a recruitment agency, or it might be one that you have arranged directly with the employer after applying for the position. The interview might take place in your home country, with the prospective employer traveling to interview nurses there, or you might travel to the United States for your interview. Interviews also may be conducted electronically, by telephone, or by **video conference.**

For any employment interview, it is very important to be on time, or even early, for the interview. You *never* should be late for an interview. Lateness, regardless of the reason, may suggest that you do not take the position (or the interview) seriously.

Phases of the Interview Process

An interview usually proceeds through three phases. In the first phase, you and the interviewer will meet and simply get to know each other.

The interview then continues into the second, or fact-finding, phase. You will have the opportunity to find out more about the position and to ask questions. This is also the interviewer's opportunity to find out more about you, probably using your résumé or portfolio as a guide and asking for clarification or more information on the facts you have presented about yourself. You should answer questions honestly and enthusiastically. In this phase of the interview, you also may have a chance to ask questions about salary and benefits.

During the final phase of the interview, the interviewer will generally explain the next steps of the hiring process and determine if you have any further questions. Before the end of the interview, be sure you thank the interviewer for his or her time and consideration. It is also a good idea to obtain his or her contact information (usually by requesting a business card) for questions you may think of later and for the purpose of writing the interviewer a thank you letter (see Appendix A for a sample thank you letter following an interview). Also, it is important that, by the end of the interview, you understand what the next steps in the process are and when you should expect to be notified of the employer's hiring decision.

Dressing for Success

It is important to dress professionally for the interview and to be well groomed. It is best to dress conservatively and also to be conservative with such things as nails, jewelry, make-up, and hair style. Men should wear a suit or a jacket with coordinated slacks, shirt, and tie. Women should wear a suit or a jacket with coordinated skirt or slacks. You should never dress casually for an interview.

Follow-Up Letter

It is always appropriate for you to send a follow-up communication after the interview, especially if you are interested in the position.

This should consist of a brief note of thanks—either handwritten or typewritten—indicating your continued interest in the position and thanking the interviewer for the opportunity to meet with him or her.

Hiring Process

A hiring decision may occur at the close of the interview, or it may occur later. If you receive an offer of employment, the salary and benefits should be made completely clear to you as a part of this offer. If you are offered the position, you might decide that you definitely want this job and that the pay and benefits are desirable, in which case you would accept the offer of employment.

Declining the Position

You may have decided that the job is not what you are looking for, in which case you would decline the offer of employment. If you feel that you are not ready to make a decision, particularly if you have other job interviews scheduled, you may need to reply to the employment offer at a later time.

Whichever decision you make, it is important to be clear, honest, and polite. You should not feel pressured to take a job if you are not sure. It is not uncommon to take several days to come to a decision about an employment offer. However, if you know the job is not right for you, then politely decline and thank the interviewer for his or her time.

Not Being Offered the Position

If you are not offered the position, you may want to ask why. This information can help you to prepare for the next time you interview for a position, or it may help you decide to focus on a different strategy for finding a job. If you find out about the rejection by mail, consider calling the employer for more information if it was not made clear in the letter.

Accepting the Position

If you accept the position, the next step in the hiring process is to agree to the salary, benefits, orientation process, and the date you will begin work. If you are moving to the United States, you also will need to make sure you understand any housing and transportation arrangements that the employer is providing. Additionally, some employers offer acculturation programs for foreign-educated nurses. It is important that you understand all of the benefits of the position before accepting it. It is also appropriate for you to request salary and benefit information in writing.

Contracts

Some employers or recruitment agencies may offer you a contract as part of the hiring process. A contract is a legally binding document that spells out the rights and obligations of the parties involved—generally, the employer and the employee. Be sure all salary, employee benefit, orientation, and other agreement details are written into the contract document. Also, make sure you understand and agree to all of your obligations as specified in the contract.

Be careful to review the contract time period if it is specified. For example, does it require you to work for 1 year or 2 years before leaving the job? Does it impose a cancellation fee that you must pay if you decide to leave earlier? Not all employers will require formal employment contracts. If there is no formal contract, you should always request a letter outlining your wages and benefits so that you have it for your records. For more information on contracts, see chapter 2, "Choosing a Recruiter."

Networking

As soon as you have accepted employment in the United States, it is important that you begin networking. Networking is a process of developing and maintaining relationships with people whose skills and experiences add to your professional well-being. The goal of networking is to identify, value, and maintain relationships with people who are sources of information, advice, and support (Kelly, 2007). Networking helps you to connect with your new workplace environment more easily, better, and faster.

Networking Opportunities

There are a variety of networking opportunities, such as seeking workplace introductions, establishing ties to the local community, and searching out professional society affiliations. After being hired, it is appropriate to ask to be introduced to people with whom you will work or to other foreign-educated nurses. It would be ideal to be introduced to nurses who work for your new manager and who have come from your particular country.

If being a part of a religious community is important to you, your employer should be able to help you find a list of religious organizations. Contacting these organizations will help you meet people who share your religious beliefs and who also will assist you in joining a new community.

Another valuable source of networking is to become involved with professional nursing associations, including state and local affiliates of ANA and specialty nursing organizations that support and promote nursing practice in a wide variety of nursing specialty practice areas, such as critical care, emergency nursing, women's health, or pediatric nursing. See chapter 11 for more information on nursing associations and other professional resources.

WORKPLACE RIGHTS AND OBLIGATIONS

As you prepare for your new position in the United States, it is important to understand that you will be expected to be a responsible and dependable employee and to comply with the policies of your new employer. These policies should be explained to you by your new employer. In addition to your obligations as an employee, you also have certain rights that are guaranteed by law to you as a U.S. worker.

Unions and Collective Bargaining

In the United States, employees have the right to join unions and to be represented by them for the purposes of bargaining for pay, benefits, working conditions, salary, and other conditions of employment (this is referred to as **collective bargaining**). The right of employees who work for nongovernment employers to join and be represented by unions is outlined by the National Labor Relations Act, which also addresses the rights, obligations, and conduct of unions and employers (National Labor Relations Board, 2009). The union representation and collective bargaining rights of nurses who work for city, county, or state hospitals or health departments are addressed in state labor laws. For nurses who work for federal health care facilities (such as those operated by the Veterans Health Administration), their rights are addressed in the Federal Labor Relations Act.

Union Representation for Nurses

ANA and several of the individual state nurses associations affiliated with ANA have provided union representation to many nurses for over 60 years. In 1946, ANA began actively working to secure the economic and general welfare of nurses. Many nurses at that time were distressed by poor working conditions and wages, and many felt that their employers were not listening to their complaints and not acting on their concerns (Foley, Williams, & Claborn, 2006).

Since then, many nurses in the United States have opted for union representation either through their state nurses associations or through "traditional" labor unions, that is, those that originated to represent workers in occupations such as service workers, teachers, truck drivers, and others. Unions representing nurses typically bargain not only on economic issues such as wages and benefits, but also on professional practice issues including staffing levels, being asked to work temporarily on unfamiliar units, participation in decision making, and other areas.

An estimated 19% of employed nurses in the United States are represented by unions. However, many unions have indicated a strong interest in organizing more nurses. You should inquire as to whether nurses in your new workplace are unionized or not and if joining the union is mandatory. In most unionized workplaces, you will be required to pay dues or a fee to the union. In some, joining or paying fees to the union is voluntary.

Antidiscrimination Laws

Many U.S. state and local laws prohibit discrimination in employment, public accommodations, and other areas of public life. Federal civil rights and equal employment opportunity laws prohibit employers from treating employees or applicants for employment differently based on a number of characteristics, including race, ethnicity, gender, national origin, religion, age, and disability. Many state and local laws also prohibit discrimination based on these characteristics. Some state and local laws may provide broader protections than federal laws, prohibiting discrimination based on additional factors not addressed in federal law, such as sexual orientation.

Federal civil rights, labor, and immigration laws include important protections that are relevant to immigrant nurses. A good summary of these is included in the *Voluntary Code of Ethical Conduct for the Recruitment of Foreign-Educated Nurses to the United States*, which is available at http://www.faitinternationalrecruitment.org.

Labor Standards

Wage and Hour Laws

Most nurses in the United States work for an hourly wage. The Fair Labor Standards Act, a federal law, requires that workers receive overtime pay when they work more than 40 hours in a week—or, in many health care facilities, when they work beyond 80 hours in a 2-week period or 8 hours in a day (U.S. Department of Labor, 2009).

Typically, overtime pay is at one and a half times the employee's regular rate of pay. Some states have their own wage and hour laws, which may be stricter than the federal requirements. Also, in hospitals in which nurses are represented by a union, the collective bargaining agreement (the union contract) may include different requirements for overtime pay.

Mandatory Overtime

In many health care facilities, employers sometimes require a nurse to remain on duty after his or her shift ends. This is referred to as **mandatory overtime**. When a nurse agrees to work beyond his or her shift—that is, when the employer does not mandate the nurse to do so—it is often referred to as **voluntary overtime.** Many nurses have complained that hospitals have utilized mandatory overtime on a routine basis to make up for staffing shortages.

ANA and many other nursing organizations oppose the use of mandatory overtime as a staffing strategy because they see it as posing risks to patients and to nurses when staff are required to work long, unplanned hours, often past the point of being fatigued (Bonczek, 2007). Legislation that prohibits mandatory overtime has been passed in some states and is being considered in others.

Employer-Provided Benefits

In addition to the salary you receive, most employers offer a benefits package to employees who work at least 20 hours per week. Some employers only offer benefits to full-time workers, generally considered to be those workers who are regularly scheduled for 40 hours per week. Benefits usually are part of a package offered to an employee upon hiring. Benefits packages vary among employers and may include some or all of the following.

Health Insurance

Health insurance covers all or part of the cost of hospitalization, medical services, and prescription medicines. In many cases, employers also provide dental benefits and vision care (eye examinations and eyeglasses). Covered services may vary significantly between employers, as may the amount of medical costs that are covered.

Most employer-provided health plans require the employee to pay some of the cost of their medical care. In addition, most plans require the employee to pay part of their health insurance premium (the fee that is paid to the health insurance company). Generally, this amount is deducted from the employee's paycheck. Some employers may require employees to pay only a small amount each month toward the cost of health insurance premiums; other employers may require more significant payments.

In most workplaces, your health insurance plan also can cover your spouse and dependent children. Most employers require you to pay an additional amount for family coverage. However, this benefit may be very useful if your spouse is not working, or is working in a job that either does not provide health insurance or provides health insurance benefits that are not as good or comprehensive as the benefits provided by your employer.

Vacation Pay

Vacation pay provides you with your regular wages during time off from work. You should inquire as to how much vacation time you will receive each year. Many employers offer an increasing amount of vacation time for continued years of service—for example, an employee may start off with 3 weeks of vacation in the first year, and this may increase to 4 weeks after 2 years of employment. Employers vary in the amount of vacation pay they provide.

Sick Pay

Sick pay provides payment, usually at your regular rate of pay, when you are ill for a brief period of time (e.g., 1 day or a few days). Employers differ in terms of how much sick time they will offer an employee and the conditions under which it can be used.

Holidays

Most employers provide employees with paid days off for specified holidays. Employers may differ in terms of which holidays they recognize for the purpose of holiday pay. Since hospitals must function every day of the year, nurses often have to work on holidays.

Many employers provide additional pay for working on a holiday. Some provide another paid day off when an employee works on a holiday, and still others offer both additional pay and another day off. In hospitals in which nurses are represented by a union, the union contract will include details on holiday pay. Table 5.1 lists the federal holidays observed in the United States.

The Uniform Holidays Bill of 1968 (taking effect in 1971) declared that official holidays are to be observed on a Monday, except for New Year's Day, Independence Day, Veterans' Day, Thanksgiving, and Christmas. In the United States, most retail businesses close on Thanksgiving and Christmas but remain open on all other holidays. Private businesses often observe only the major holidays (New Year's Day, Memorial Day, Independence Day, Labor Day, Thanksgiving, and Christmas). Some also add the Friday after Thanksgiving, or one or more of the other federal holidays.

Retirement Benefits

Retirement benefits provide an employee with an income when he or she retires from employment. Most employees who retire qualify for Social Security benefits from the federal government (see section on Social Security later in this chapter), but these benefits are generally modest (the maximum benefit amount in 2009 is $2,323 per month, so retirement plans provide an important additional source of income for retirees).

Traditionally, in the United States, retirement plans provided a specific amount of income to an employee after retirement—calculated either as a specific dollar amount or as a percentage of the employee's preretirement salary. Today, many employers have moved away from offering such plans, instead offering employees the opportunity to put a percentage of their salary into a fund on which they can draw following retirement. Many employers, as part of their benefits package, pay a specified amount of money into the employee's retirement fund as well. These retirement funds are commonly referred to as 401(k) plans or 503(b) plans.

Table 5.1

TRADITIONAL HOLIDAYS IN THE UNITED STATES

DATE	OFFICIAL NAME	REMARKS
January 1st	New Year's Day	First day of the year.
Third Monday in January	Martin Luther King Day	Honors Martin Luther King, civil rights leader. A day devoted to volunteering in the community.
Third Monday in February	Washington's Birthday or Presidents' Day	Traditionally honors the first President of the United States, George Washington. In recent years, has been known as Presidents' Day to honor all U.S. Presidents.
Last Monday in May	Memorial Day	Honors the nation's war dead from the Civil War forward; marks the unofficial beginning of the summer season.
July 4th	Independence Day or the 4th of July	Celebrates the signing of the U.S. Declaration of Independence.
First Monday in September	Labor Day	Celebrates the achievements of workers and the labor movement; marks the unofficial end of the summer season.
Second Monday in October	Columbus Day	Honors Christopher Columbus, traditional discoverer of the Americas. In some areas, also a celebration of Native American culture.
November 11th	Veterans Day	Honors all veterans of the U.S. Armed Forces.
Fourth Thursday in November	Thanksgiving Day	Traditionally celebrates the giving of thanks for the autumn harvest—also the giving of thanks for one's family and possessions.
December 25th	Christmas Day	Celebrates the Nativity of Jesus. Some people consider aspects of this religious holiday, such as giving gifts and decorating a Christmas tree, to be secular rather than explicitly Christian.

While you may be many years away from retirement, you should start contributing to the plan your employer offers as soon as you are eligible to do so, especially if the employer's contribution is dependent on the percentage you contribute.

Other Benefits

Other benefits offered by an employer may include such things as:

- Life insurance, which provides a specified amount of money to a surviving spouse or other family member (or, usually, anyone else the employee designates) upon the employee's death;
- Accidental death and dismemberment insurance, which pays a specified amount of money if the employee dies or suffers a major injury as the result of an accident; and
- Long-term disability insurance, which provides a regular income (usually a percentage of the employee's salary) if an employee becomes unable to work because of injury or disability.

Family and Medical Leave Act

Employers are required by the federal Family and Medical Leave Act (FMLA) to allow up to 12 weeks of unpaid leave during any 12-month period to care for a newborn or newly adopted child, to care for an immediate family member with a serious health condition, or to take medical leave when the employee is unable to work because of a serious health condition.

Some states may require employers to provide more family and medical leave than is required by federal law. Many employers also provide more generous family and medical leave benefits. For example, although the FMLA only requires employers to grant unpaid leave, some employers will provide employees with paid parental leave for the birth or adoption of a child. In addition, union contracts may require the employer to provide greater benefits than are required by federal law.

Government-Provided Benefits

Some benefits for employees (or retired employees) are financed at least in part by employers but are made available through government.

Social Security

Social Security provides a monthly payment to older retirees. Depending on when an employee was born, the age at which she or he can receive full benefits ranges from 65 to 67. Social Security also may be available to individuals who are no longer able to work because of a permanent disability.

Social Security is funded by a payroll tax (paid in addition to federal and state income taxes); the employer and employee each contribute 6.2% of the employee's income to help finance the system. In order to qualify to receive benefits, an employee must have paid into the system for 40 quarters (the equivalent of 10 years).

Medicare

Medicare is a federal program that provides health insurance to individuals who: (1) are at least 65 years of age, (2) have End-Stage Renal Disease, or (3) are permanently disabled and have been receiving Social Security benefits for at least 2 years. Like Social Security, Medicare is financed by a payroll tax—the employer and employee each contribute 1.45% of the employee's income.

Workers' Compensation

Workers' compensation is a program that provides medical treatment and other benefits for an employee who is injured at work. It also provides income for workers who are disabled and unable to work because of an on-the-job injury. State laws specify employers' requirements for participating in and providing benefits under this program, which is generally financed by employers.

WORKPLACE HAZARDS

There are laws that protect employees from workplace hazards in U.S. employment. The Occupational Safety and Health Act (OSHA) of 1970 helps to ensure healthful and safe working conditions in the

U.S. workplace. The law requires isolation procedures for patients with highly contagious diseases, radiation safety guidelines for x-ray and nuclear equipment, proper grounding of electrical equipment, protective storage of flammable and combustible liquids, and the gloving of all personnel when handling bodily fluids.

Employers are expected to ensure that gloves and necessary equipment are present in the workplace to prevent exposure to infectious diseases. You may find that the concept of wearing gloves for many routine nursing procedures may be different from what you have previously experienced in other countries. Additionally, handwashing procedures in the United States are extremely strict due to the prevalent transmission of infections between patients. The use of gowns, goggles, and masks also is widespread, as are personal protective devices.

Safe Needle Devices

As a new nurse in the U.S. health care system, be sure to inquire about the use of safe needle devices to protect yourself from bloodborne diseases and needle stick injuries. In 2000, the ANA was part of an effort to pass national legislation that expanded the use of safe needle devices, such as retractable needles and other types of safe needles that prevent needle sticks and subsequent exposure.

Preventing Physical Injuries

More OSHA standards were issued in 2000 to protect employees from musculoskeletal injuries that are caused when there is a physical mismatch between the physical ability of the worker and the physical demands of the workplace. One example of common injuries in nursing practice is back injuries resulting from lifting patients.

It was once thought that teaching nurses proper body mechanics to lift and to turn patients resulted in fewer injuries. However, back injuries may have many causes. Because of this, the ANA now recommends the use of assistive patient-handling devices for lifting, transferring, and turning patients. In May 2005, one state legislature in the United States passed the first legislation that encourages the availability and use of assistive patient-handling devices (Ahrens, 2006).

PROFESSIONAL WORKPLACE PRACTICE

When nurses experience dissatisfaction with the U.S. nursing workplace, it generally is centered on the absence of professional autonomy and accountability. Magnet hospitals have demonstrated that governance structures that include nurse autonomy and accountability are responsible for attracting and retaining the best nurses; the best nurses provide the best patient care. Magnet characteristics have now been regarded as having affected not only the quality of the workplace, but also the quality of patient care (Mancini, 2007).

Governance Structures

Shared or self-governance structures, described earlier in this chapter, are sometimes referred to as professional workplace practice models. Such models are built upon the foundation of the professional workplace instead of the organizational hierarchy. There is a sharing of responsibility for decision making between those nurses who are in management roles and those nurses who are involved in direct patient care. Such models seek to change nurses' positions from dependent employees to independent, accountable professionals (Mancini, 2007). These models are prevalent in hospitals that have been designated with Magnet recognition.

Nursing Theories

Other professional workplace practice models are built around a specific nursing theory, and there are several nursing theorists who have constructed theories of nursing practice. Theories of nursing are created around metaparadigms, or large concepts. The four prevailing metaparadigms in nursing are: nursing, person, health, and environment. The nursing theorists suggest relationships between and among the metaparadigms (Sullivan, 2006).

Some nursing service organizations within U.S. workplace settings have adopted one of the nursing theories and have built policies, procedures, and practices to be congruent with the theory. Some models may combine theory-based practice and self- or shared governance.

As you interview for a nursing position in the United States, you should inquire about the presence and type of professional workplace practice model in that institution. Such structures help to create a satisfying professional workplace.

INTERNATIONAL RIGHTS

The General Assembly of the United Nations adopted the Universal Declaration of Human Rights on December 10, 1948. The intention was that these international rights be disseminated throughout the world and that human rights be the rule of law in all nations, in all parts of the world.

Article 2 of the declaration states, "Everyone is entitled to all the rights and freedoms set forth in this Declaration, without distinction of any kind, such as race, color, sex, language, religion, political or other opinion, national or social origin, property, birth or other status. Furthermore, no distinction shall be made on the basis of the political, jurisdictional or international status of the country or territory to which a person belongs, whether it be independent, trust, non-self-governing or under any other limitation of sovereignty." The clear intent of this article is that all persons in the world are recognized as having all the rights and freedoms without distinction based on any of the cited variables, whether based on personal, political, or country-of-origin considerations.

Article 6 of the declaration states, "Everyone has the right to recognition everywhere as a person before the law." This article states the intent that every person has rights everywhere, in all countries.

Article 7 of the international rights declaration states, "All are equal before the law and are entitled without any discrimination to equal protection of the law. All are entitled to equal protection against any discrimination in violation of this Declaration and against any incitement to such discrimination." The intent of this article is that all persons are entitled to being treated equally in all parts of the world.

Articles 23, 24, and 25 speak directly to employment and social services availability as well as security standards throughout the world. Article 23 states: (1) "Everyone has the right to work, to free choice of employment, to just and favorable conditions of work and to protection against unemployment. (2) Everyone, without any discrimination, has the right to equal pay for equal work. (3) Everyone who works has the right to just and favorable remuneration ensuring for himself and his family an existence worthy of human dignity, and supplemented, if necessary, by other means of social protection. (4) Everyone has the right to form and to join trade unions for the protection of his interests."

Article 24 states: "Everyone has the right to rest and leisure, including reasonable limitation of working hours and periodic holidays with pay."

Article 25 states: (1) "Everyone has the right to a standard of living adequate for the health and well-being of himself and of his family, including food, clothing, housing and medical care and necessary social services, and the right to security in the event of unemployment, sickness, disability, widowhood, old age or other lack of livelihood in circumstances beyond his control" (United Nations, 2008).

It is very clear that labor laws in the United States were written in **congruence** with international rights as identified by the United Nations. All U.S. labor laws are directly pertinent to, and provide protection for, U.S. citizens and those who are legal immigrants.

SUMMARY

Employment as a nurse in the United States can be a rich and rewarding experience when you select employment that meets your needs and matches your skills and qualifications. The United States is a nation of immigrants, people who came to this country from other parts of the world, and the descendents of immigrants. Laws that protect the U.S. worker provide protection for U.S. citizens and legal immigrants from all over the world. International rights for nurses who are legal immigrants from any country in the world are protected by U.S. law.

REFERENCES

Ahrens, S. (2006). Workplace issues. In J. Zerwekh & J. C. Claborn (Eds.). *Nursing today: Transition and trends* (5th ed.). St. Louis: Saunders.

Bonczek, M. E. (2007). Staffing and scheduling. In P. S. Yoder Wise (Ed.), *Leading and managing in nursing* (4th ed.). St. Louis: Mosby.

Bureau of Health Professions. (2004). *National sample survey of registered nurses.* Retrieved January 29, 2009, from http://www.bhpr.hrsa.gov/healthworkforce/rnsurvey04/2.htm

Davis, C. R. (2005). International migration: Easing the transition to practice. In P. Kritek (Ed.), *Building global alliances II: The evolving health care migration* (pp. 33–36). Philadelphia: CGFNS.

Foley, M., Williams, K., & Claborn, J. C. (2006). Collective bargaining: Traditional and non-traditional approaches. In J. Zerwekh & J. C. Claborn (Eds.), *Nursing today: Transition and trends* (5th ed.). St. Louis: Saunders.

Kelly, K. (2007). Power, politics and influence. In P. S. Yoder Wise (Ed.), *Leading and managing in nursing* (4th ed.). St. Louis: Mosby.

Kramer, M., & Schmalenberg, C. (2004). Development and evaluation of essentials of magnetism tool. *Journal of Nursing Administration, 34,* 365–378.

Mancini, M. E. (2007). Understanding and designing organizational structures. In P. S. Yoder-Wise (Ed.), *Leading and managing in nursing* (4th ed.). St. Louis: Mosby.

National Labor Relations Board. (2009). *What is the National Labor Relations Act?* Retrieved January 30, 2009, fromhttp://www.nlrb.gov/Workplace_Rights/i_am_new_to_this_website/what_is_the_national_labor_relations_act.aspx

Sullivan, A. (2006). Nursing theory. In J. Zerwekh & J. C. Claborn (Eds.), *Nursing today: Transition and trends* (5th ed.). St. Louis: Saunders.

United Nations. (2008). Universal Declaration of Human Rights. Retrieved October 29, 2008, from http://www.un.org/Overview/rights.html

U.S. Department of Labor. (2009). *Compliance Assistance—Fair Labor Standards Act (FLSA).* Retrieved January 30, 2009, from http://www.dol.gov/esa/whd/flsa

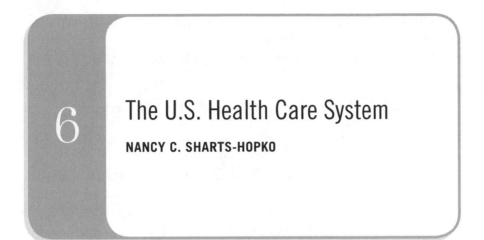

6

The U.S. Health Care System

NANCY C. SHARTS-HOPKO

In This Chapter

Organization of the Health Care System

Health Care Financing

Recent Trends in Health Care

Quality and Safety in Health Care

Access to Health Care Information

Alternative Health Practices

Summary

Keywords

Alternative therapies: Therapeutic or preventive health care practices, such as homeopathy, naturopathy, chiropractic, and herbal medicine, that complement conventional medical methods.

Biomedical research: Medical research and evaluation of new treatments for both safety and efficacy in what are termed clinical trials, and all other research that contributes to the development of new treatments.

Botanicals: Drugs or products made directly from plants.

Centers for Medicare and Medicaid Services (CMS): The federal agency responsible for administering the Medicare, Medicaid, SCHIP (State Children's Health Insurance), HIPAA (Health Insurance Portability and Accountability Act), and CLIA (Clinical Laboratory Improvement Amendments) programs and several other health-related programs. Formerly known as the Health Care Financing Administration (HCFA).

Community-based care: Services provided in one's own home or other community settings; a variety of health care options that allow people to stay in their homes, while still providing important health care support.

Coordinated care: Includes strategies to make health care systems more cost-effective and responsive to the needs of people with complex chronic illnesses.

Curative care: Refers to treatment and therapies provided to a patient with intent to improve symptoms and cure the patient's medical problem.

Disaster preparedness: Process of ensuring that an organization is prepared in the event of a forecasted disaster to minimize loss of life, injury, and damage to property and can provide rescue, relief, rehabilitation, and other services after the disaster.

Hospice: A usually small residential institution for terminally ill patients where treatment focuses on the patient's well-being rather than a cure and includes drugs for pain management and often spiritual counseling.

Meals on Wheels: Provides home-delivered meals to people in need, usually the elderly or the disabled.

Municipal hospitals: Hospitals controlled by city government.

Palliative care: A specialized form of care focused on the pain, symptoms, and stress of serious illness.

Whether you are considering coming to the United States for employment or you already have begun the visa and licensure processes, understanding the scope and structure of the U.S. health care system can be a daunting task for foreign-educated nurses. Nurses who have basic knowledge of the way health services are organized in the United States will be better able to function competently and to help patients and families navigate through the system's many channels. The purpose of this chapter is to provide you with an understanding of how health care decisions are made, both economically and organizationally, by physicians, other health care providers, patients, and their families.

ORGANIZATION OF THE HEALTH CARE SYSTEM

In the United States, individuals access health care services through a complex array of public or private clinics, private practices, commercial walk-in settings, employee or school health services, urgent care settings, and hospital systems. The system is large, with over 7,500 hospitals, 2.4 million registered nurses, and 560,000 physicians (Bureau of Labor Statistics, 2008).

Public Versus Private Health Care

The U.S. health care system includes large numbers of both public and private health care providers. *Public* sources of health care are directly managed and funded by a government agency. They include federal, state, county, and **municipal hospitals** and clinics. Examples of services provided by the federal government include those of the Veterans Health Administration, which cares for former active duty military personnel, and the Indian Health Service, which provides care to those who live on Native American tribal lands. Other examples include city and county hospitals such as Bellevue Hospital Center and other hospitals in the New York City Health and Hospitals Corporation, San Francisco General Hospital, Los Angeles County–University of Southern California (USC) Medical Center, and Cook County Stroger Hospital in Chicago.

Public clinics and hospitals provide care primarily for lower-income individuals and families. The system of publicly provided care has diminished over the past 30 years as many governments shifted away from direct provision of services to contracting with insurance companies to provide services through private hospitals. While public clinics and hospitals can and do charge for their services, they usually are heavily funded by tax dollars.

Private sources of health care include not-for-profit and for-profit clinics, practices, and hospitals. Not-for-profit hospitals and clinics charge for services and receive insurance reimbursement for care, but they do not expect to make a profit. All revenue beyond their expenses is to be used for the benefit of the organization. For-profit entities, on the other hand, are operated to generate profits for private owners or shareholders.

Primary, Secondary, and Tertiary Care

In the United States, the level of health care is designated as primary, secondary, or tertiary. These terms refer both to the acuity of care that is provided as well as the nature and location of that care.

Primary Care

The Institute of Medicine (IOM, 1994) defines primary care as "care that is accessible, comprehensive, coordinated, continuous, and accountable." Primary care providers include physicians, nurse practitioners, and physician assistants. Ideally they provide care for people over time that includes health promotion and prevention, the management of acute illnesses or injuries, and the management of chronic conditions. The primary care provider is the point of referral for inpatient or specialty services.

Secondary Care

Primary care providers refer people with complex problems to specialists, or secondary care providers, for their greater, more specific expertise. Common examples include medical specialties such as ophthalmology or dermatology, or nonroutine services such as physical therapy.

Tertiary Care

Tertiary care is advanced or complex care that is provided by medical specialists in referral centers—often academic medical centers that have strong programs of research and facilities designed for specialized diagnostic and treatment procedures.

Managed Care

Managed care refers to a system of care that became widespread in the United States beginning in 1973 with passage of the Health Maintenance Organization Act, which is federal legislation that was intended to help reduce health care costs. Originally, managed care referred to the enrollment of people in health maintenance organizations (HMOs), a system or network of health care providers and services that encompassed all levels of care. These HMOs sought to contain costs by ordering bulk purchases of goods and services; limiting diagnostic tests, prescriptions, and referrals to specialty service providers; and using incentives for people to reduce their illness risks by incorporating healthy lifestyle changes and using early screening and other preventive services.

Role of Insurance Providers

Today, most health insurance companies operate using managed care approaches, in which insurers contract with health care providers, such as physicians and nurse practitioners, who agree to operate within the insurer's financial parameters. Most managed care organizations require patients to select their primary care provider from a list approved by the insurance company. This listing of approved providers is called the insurer's "network."

In many managed care plans, primary care providers function as "gatekeepers," meaning that a patient is required to get a referral from his or her primary care provider (and, in many cases, approval from the managed care plan) before seeing a specialist. While these requirements were intended to reduce unnecessary use of specialist services, many people feel that they result in additional time and expense as well as in reduced access to services. In recent years, many managed care plans have loosened or eliminated some of their requirements for referrals or prior approval for specialist visits.

When using a managed care plan for in-patient hospital care, the patient is restricted to using only hospitals and providers within the insurer's network. If the patient selects a provider or hospital that is not "in-network," the patient pays additional costs. This occurs because the insurance companies contract with certain providers and hospitals that agree to accept reimbursement at a lower, negotiated rate.

Public Health

Public health services are directed at communities and populations for the prevention, management, or elimination of disease and for health promotion. Disease surveillance and vaccination programs, health education for risk reduction, food safety oversight, and the operation of sexually transmitted disease clinics are examples of common public health strategies in the United States.

Centers for Disease Control and Prevention

Since the World Trade Center attacks in 2001 and Hurricane Katrina in 2005, local and state health departments have increasingly focused on planning and preparedness for natural or man-made disasters. Nationally, the Centers for Disease Control and Prevention (CDC), an agency within the U.S. Department of Health and Human Services (HHS), plays a leading role in coordinating and funding public health activities, including **disaster preparedness** efforts.

The CDC monitors the health, illness, and injury of the U.S. population; advocates for national health policies focused on health promotion and disease prevention; and promotes health education. The program units within CDC address workplace health and safety, infectious disease management, terrorism and emergency preparedness, environmental health, health promotion, health information, and global health (CDC, 2008a).

Environmental Health

Within the field of public health, the practice of environmental health has grown significantly in the past several years. Health care providers and health care institutions are increasingly attentive to their impact on the environment. Whether to use disposable versus recyclable equipment is now more than a cost concern; it has become an environmental consideration. How toxic or infectious substances, including medications, are disposed of is a concern because of their potential for contaminating the food and water supply or for spreading infection.

The international coalition *Health Care Without Harm* has been formed to sensitize health care workers to the need to address pollution by the health care industry. One example of the coalition's work is its agenda of eradicating the use, and safely disposing, of mercury thermometers (Health Care Without Harm, 2008).

Ambulatory Care

Ambulatory care is health care delivered outside of an inpatient or residential setting. Ambulatory care settings include physician, nurse practitioner and dental practices, hospital outpatient clinics, community clinics, school and employee health centers, and urgent care centers.

Urgent Care Centers

Urgent care centers are walk-in (or ambulatory care) facilities usually operating for extended hours where people can be treated for acute illnesses and injuries that are beyond the scope of a primary care provider. There are over 8,000 urgent care facilities in the United States, and their appeal is the accessibility of care as well as the favorable cost compared to hospital emergency department visits (Urgent Care Association of America, 2008). The CDC estimates that over 80% of emergency department visits do not require that level of care; urgent care is filling a gap in the health care system.

Walk-In Clinics

A more recent trend is the emergence of walk-in clinics in commercial venues, such as discount stores or pharmacies. Also referred to as convenient care clinics, retail clinics and minute clinics, they offer a limited range of primary care services that are more convenient, and typically less expensive, than a visit to a primary care provider's office or an emergency department. They are usually staffed by nurse practitioners, although physician assistants and physicians also work in these sites.

Ambulatory or Day Surgery

Ambulatory surgery can be defined as any surgical procedure that does not require an overnight stay in the hospital. At this time, about 65% of all surgical procedures performed in the United States are performed on a same-day basis.

While the original impetus for this trend was cost savings, there are additional benefits. The risk of hospital-acquired infection is reduced when people return quickly to their homes from a hospital environment, and people tend to recover more quickly in a familiar environment. The technology that has enabled procedures to be performed as same-day procedures is less invasive, so the healing that is required is lessened. Patients are monitored for a few hours after their procedure—typically until they are awake, have stable vital signs, are able to tolerate oral fluids, and can urinate. Day surgery requires that patients and their family members receive clear instructions for post-operative care and symptoms that require immediate attention. It is common for a nurse or surgeon to call patients within a few hours or days of discharge to monitor their status.

Home Care and Community-Based Care

Home care is care provided in the home by health care workers. Most commonly health care professionals, such as nurses or physical therapists, monitor and manage care on a daily to weekly basis. Nurses may perform procedures such as changing intravenous lines, while routine daily care may be provided by home health aides or by family members. The rise in home care has accompanied the reduction in hospital admissions and hospital lengths of stay. Health care agencies that provide home care are eligible for certification by The Joint Commission, the same agency that certifies hospitals (The Joint Commission, 2008), or by the Community Health Accreditation Program (http://www.chapinc.org). Another term that is used when health care services are provided in the patient's home is **community-based care.** Community-based care provides a variety of health care options that allows people to stay in their homes, while still providing important health care support.

Hospice Care

Hospice care is professional support for individuals and their families who face a life-threatening illness, usually terminal or end-stage (Hospicenet, 2008). Hospice care may be provided in hospital settings, but it is more commonly provided in the patient's home or in a home-like setting. Hospice care is based on the principle that death is a normal part of life, and quality of life while a person is dying is a paramount value. Moreover, people who are dying and their family members should be treated compassionately and with dignity.

Hospice care is authorized when the provider indicates that death is imminent or expected within a certain time frame. Care is provided by a team including a physician, a nurse, a chaplain or other spiritual advisor, if desired, and other team members as needed. The management of symptoms such as pain, dyspnea, and anxiety is a primary concern, and spiritual care is often a significant part of hospice care.

Care is planned in accordance with the patient's wishes and the family's needs.

Family members are likely to be the primary day-to-day caregivers, while health professionals ensure that they have the knowledge and resources they need to allow their family member to die as comfortably and as peacefully as possible. The hospice team can refer family members to resources for bereavement support following the patient's death.

Long-Term Care

Long-term care refers to a variety of medical and nonmedical services to people with a chronic illness or disability (Medicare, 2008a). Most long-term care is provided to assist people with activities of daily living such as eating, dressing, bathing, or going to the bathroom. Long-term care is not age-specific or place-specific. People with temporary or permanent disabilities at any age may require long-term care. Most of the time, the term is used in association with care for elderly persons.

In 2007, 9 million individuals required long-term care; by 2010, it is estimated that 12 million older adults will require this service. The U.S. Department of Health and Human Services, which administers Medicare, estimates that among adults who reach the age of 65, 40% will enter a nursing home, and 10% will be there for 5 or more years. As noted previously, this is a dauntingly expensive proposition. As Medicare describes long-term care, the options range from community-based services to home health, including senior or disabled housing, assisted living, continuing or life-care communities, and nursing homes, to name a few.

Community-Based Services

Community-based services include free or low-cost services that help older adults remain safely and healthily in their homes. These can include adult day care, senior centers, **Meals on Wheels,** financial guidance and assistance with filing taxes, case management, and daily telephone reassurance.

Some older adults may move in with a family member, or conversely, rent space in their homes to an individual who will in return provide some daily assistance. Senior or disabled housing is available, and these facilities are often publicly subsidized so that the resident pays only a portion of the monthly cost. Residents live in their own apartments and typically have services such as laundry, shopping, or housekeeping available.

Assisted Living

Assisted living is a costlier approach to long-term care than community-based services. Residents typically live in their own apartment within a complex and have available such options as assistance with activities of daily living and group meals. Social and recreational activities are commonly provided. On-site health care services also may be available. The cost of assisted living can range widely—up to many thousands of dollars a month for a large apartment in an expensive part of the country. Neither long-term care nor Medicare contributes to the costs of assisted care.

Continuing Care Retirement Communities

Continuing care retirement communities, or life-care communities, offer levels of care as the resident needs them. A healthy older person or a couple might move into an apartment or cottage and live totally independently. Later, the person or couple might require assisted living. Finally, the person will move into the nursing home associated with the community. This is an expensive option. Medicare reports that in 2004 entry fees ranged from $38,000 to $400,000 and the monthly fee ranged from $650 to $3,500 (Medicare, 2008a). Long-term care and Medicare will not contribute to costs associated with continuing care retirement communities. Residents often sign over their homes and other assets to fund their residency at such facilities.

Nursing Homes

Nursing homes provide a wide range of personal care and health services, such as activities of daily living for people with a variety of physical, emotional, or cognitive problems. Individuals must fund this care privately or with special insurance because Medicare does not cover this aspect of nursing home care.

Medicare does pay for time-limited skilled nursing care after an illness or injury, and, depending on the facility, Medicaid will cover nursing home costs after an individual's personal assets are spent. In general, it is more likely that individuals will be able to use Medicaid to remain in the setting after their funds are exhausted if it is a nonprofit entity.

Continuing care retirement communities, as well as nursing homes, can be operated as voluntary, nonprofit, or for-profit organizations. Many nonprofit facilities are affiliated with religious groups.

HEALTH CARE FINANCING

In many countries, both private and public sources of health insurance are used. That is the case in the United States, but what is unique in this country is that private insurance is dominant (Chua, 2006). In 2003, 62% of nonelderly Americans had private employer-sponsored insurance, 5% purchased private insurance individually, 15% were insured by public programs such as Medicaid, and 18% were uninsured. Nearly all people age 65 and older are insured through the public program Medicare.

Private Employer-Sponsored Insurance

Private employer-sponsored insurance has been a mainstay of employee benefits since World War II. Employers contract with insurance companies to offer a specific coverage package in which employees can either participate or not. Employees pay some portion of the insurance costs, particularly as they enroll other family members in the plan. The benefits that are covered vary across employers; for instance, some employers provide dental or vision coverage while others do not.

Individual Insurance

Individuals can purchase health insurance directly from insurance companies—the cost is completely born by the individual subscriber in this case. The cost of health insurance varies widely depending on the insurance company; the scope of benefits the individual seeks; and the person's age, health status, and presence of known health risk factors or preexisting conditions (diagnoses that existed in the past or exist at the time the person seeks health insurance).

Medicare

Medicare is a federal insurance program that covers the health care costs of people age 65 and older as well as some people with disabilities. Medicare is financed through taxes as well as individual premiums for certain benefits. Medicare Part A covers hospitalization costs and requires no premium co-pay. People may enroll in additional coverage, for which they pay premiums. Medicare Part B covers physician services; Medicare Part C is administered through Health Management Organizations (HMOs) and is referred to as Medicare Advantage; and Medicare Part D is the recently implemented drug plan.

While Medicare has been successful in ensuring access to care for older and disabled Americans, there are gaps in coverage, including incomplete nursing home and health prevention coverage. On average, older individuals spend about 22% of their income on health-related costs despite having Medicare.

Medicaid

Medicaid is a joint federal and state program that provides insurance to many lower-income individuals. Although the federal government provides much of the funding and sets basic criteria for services and coverage, each state administers its own Medicaid program, and thus both covered services and eligibility criteria vary from state to state.

The State Children's Health Insurance Program

The State Children's Health Insurance Program (S-CHIP) was initiated in 1997 to extend coverage to children in low-income families who do not qualify for Medicaid. Like Medicaid, it is jointly funded by federal and state governments and is administered by each state.

Veterans Health Administration

The Veterans Health Administration (VHA) provides health care to veterans of the U.S. armed forces. In general, care is supposed to be provided free or at low cost for conditions directly related to individuals' military service. In reality, many veterans rely on the VHA system for all or most of their care, generally in hospitals and clinics operated directly by the VHA.

Health Care Reform

Numerous solutions have been proposed to address the major issues facing the U.S. health system—providing access to care for all Americans, controlling health care costs, and ensuring quality. Some proposals focus on market-based approaches, such as providing financial incentives to encourage more uninsured Americans to purchase health insurance. Other proposals emphasize greater direct government involvement to ensure universal coverage.

A comprehensive proposal for health reform was proposed to the U.S. Congress by President Bill Clinton in 1993, but after contentious national debate, Congress failed to pass any reform proposals. In the years since then, different approaches have been suggested by political leaders and by organizations representing physicians, nurses, hospitals, insurers, and others. With the election of President Obama, health reform again has been deemed a national political priority.

RECENT TRENDS IN HEALTH CARE

Health care in the United States is provided in a variety of settings by a team of professionals. Depending on the patient's needs, the team may include nurses, advanced practice nurses, physicians, medical social workers, speech therapists, physical therapists, occupational therapists, nutritionists, chaplains, and other specialized professionals. Traditionally the physician was in charge of a patient's care; now, particularly with the advent of managed care, the team works collaboratively, and it may be a case manager working in the health care institution or the patient's health insurance company who oversees the patient's progress through the system or through the illness episode.

While it is impossible to anticipate the future of health care in a rapidly changing environment, several trends in the United States are worth noting: the demographic shift leading to large numbers of older individuals needing health care; the impact of chronic illness and the obesity epidemic on health care delivery; the growing sensitivity to the need for **palliative care** (symptom management) particularly at the end of life; a resurgence in direct provision of health care by employers; and the emergence of concierge care.

Demographic Shift

First and foremost, worldwide there is a demographic shift as life spans increase. In wealthy, industrialized nations, we are faced with the retirement of the "baby boom" generation, the individuals who were born between approximately 1946 and 1965, after World War II. In the United States, this is the largest group in our nation's history and nearly double the size of the next generation to follow. Because of the size of the baby boom generation, the United States will experience an increasing demand for health care services by older adults—along with a shortage in the labor force available to provide care for them.

Increase in Chronic Illness and Obesity

Chronic illnesses, such as heart disease, stroke, cancer, and diabetes, are among the most prevalent, costly, and preventable of all health problems in the United States—and their incidence is expected to grow (CDC, 2008b). The prolonged course of illness and disability from such chronic diseases can result in a decreased quality of life and an increased use of health care resources. The impact of HIV/AIDS on the minority community and women also will tax the system.

In addition, the U.S. obesity epidemic has many health care implications ranging from anticipated financial demands on the system to physical demands on providers working with larger numbers of obese patients. As of 2006, over one-third of U.S. men and women are obese, and the prevalence of obesity in children is increasing (CDC, 2008c). This will not only exacerbate the incidence of chronic disease, but in the case of childhood obesity, it will also decrease the age of onset of these diseases. It will be an enormous challenge not only to provide services that are needed, but also to control health care costs as this likely scenario unfolds.

Increase in Palliative Care

There is growing sensitivity to the need to shift from **curative care** to palliative care (symptom management) at the end of life. The emergence of intensive care units in the United States in the 1960s led to an explosion of technology—and to its pervasiveness and daily use in health care settings. However, research in recent years has confirmed that patients and families desire compassionate and peaceful deaths without many technological interventions.

A number of organizations have formed to advocate on behalf of people who are dying and their families; one example is a coalition of health care systems, the *Supportive Care Coalition* (2008). This organization seeks to foster holistic, **coordinated care** for terminally ill people, to enable those who want to die in their homes to do so, and to diminish the incidence of elders dying in intensive care settings. Fortunately, there seems to be a trend toward promoting palliative care.

Employer-Provided Care

Employer-provided, on-site health care was commonplace before the emergence of managed care and the growth in litigation of the 1970s and 1980s. On-site employee health services are once again emerging as a convenient, low-cost strategy for improving employee health and curtailing overhead costs associated with health care. Moreover, this strategy addresses the needs—which may affect productivity—of employees who decline the company health insurance plan because they cannot afford their portion of the premiums. Companies that have successfully provided on-site care include Coca Cola, Goldman

Sachs, Toyota, and Novartis, among others (Corporate Research Group, 2008).

Concierge Health Care

Concierge health care, also referred to as boutique care, is controversial because it targets affluent individuals. It is the payment of an annual retainer to a primary care physician, ranging from $50 to $20,000 per family member per year, in return for which he or she will be available to the client at all times. Wait times are reduced, visits are longer, care is more individualized, house calls are available, and some practitioners will accompany their patients to specialists.

The concept emerged out of physician dissatisfaction with managed care and the extreme limitation on their time with each patient—an average per visit of as few as 7 minutes. Hospital attitudes toward concierge care have ranged from regarding it as ethically unacceptable to seizing it as economic opportunity. While many people in the health care industry have ethical concerns with the concept of concierge care, in essence, it does not differ from the already existing opportunity for people to buy expensive and inclusive health care insurance or to pay cash for luxury care—both of which are fully accepted in the U.S. health care system. Data on health outcomes associated with concierge care is not yet available.

QUALITY AND SAFETY IN HEALTH CARE

In 1998, the IOM, composed of respected national leaders in health care, launched an initiative to highlight concerns about safety and quality of health care in the United States. This initiative captured the nation's attention when it reported that as many as 98,000 people die in U.S. hospitals each year due to health care error (IOM, 1999). Other researchers have estimated that U.S. hospital deaths due to error could be as much as five times higher than the IOM's estimate (see, e.g., Zhan & Miller, 2003). Needless to say, these reports and others like them have received attention from consumers, government entities, and the health care industry.

Agency for Healthcare Research and Quality

The Agency for Healthcare Research and Quality (AHRQ, 2008) is the governmental entity within the Department of Health and Human Services charged specifically with promoting health care quality, safety, and effectiveness. AHRQ's efforts have included funding research on improving patient safety and quality, promoting the use of health information technology, and advancing evidence-based practice.

Institute for Healthcare Improvement

To hasten the movement to improve health care quality, the Institute for Healthcare Improvement (IHI) launched the 100,000 Lives Campaign in December 2004 (Berwick, Calkins, McCannon, & Hackbarth, 2006). The nation's hospitals were invited to enroll with a goal that each hospital implement six highly feasible interventions based on published evidence. The six interventions included: deploying rapid response teams with critical care expertise to respond to all codes; following published guidelines from the American College of Cardiology and the American Heart Association in caring for people with acute myocardial infarctions; reconciling medications at each and every transition in a given patient's site of care; following the CDC guidelines for prevention of central line infection; following the CDC guidelines for prevention of surgical site infections; and following the CDC guidelines for prevention of ventilator-associated pneumonia. None of these strategies represent care that is technologically challenging. By July 2006, 50% more hospitals had enrolled than anticipated, and over 123,000 lives had been saved. As a result of the initial success, IHI then launched a campaign to save 5 million lives in the 2006–2008 biennium (Institute for Healthcare Improvement, 2008).

The Centers for Medicare and Medicaid Services

In July 2008, the **Centers for Medicare and Medicaid Services (CMS)** announced that Medicare and Medicaid would no longer cover costs associated with several types of preventable harmful events, including stage III and IV pressure ulcers, falls and trauma involving nursing home or hospital patients, surgical site infections after certain procedures, vascular catheter associated infections, catheter associated urinary tract infections, administration of incompatible blood, air embolism, or unintended retention of a foreign object after surgery (Centers for Medicare and Medicaid Services [CMS], 2008). The intent behind this policy is that avoiding the costs associated with these events will motivate health care systems to institute measures to reduce their occurrence.

Corporate Quality and Safety

One initiative for improving quality and safety has come from the corporate, non–health care sector. The Leapfrog Group is an organization of large companies that purchase employee health insurance. These companies came together in 1998 in order to use their purchasing power on behalf of patient safety and health care quality. The Leapfrog Group specifically advocates four practices to improve quality and cost-efficiency of care: use of electronic health records, use of evidence-based hospital referrals, staffing intensive care units with physicians specializing in intensive care, and evaluating hospital performance on 30 patient safety indicators endorsed by the National Quality Forum (The Leapfrog Group, 2008).

Electronic Health Records

One of the great hopes for reducing health care errors is the widespread implementation of information technology. For example, many patient safety experts have advocated the use of computerized physician order entry to reduce medication errors, including errors associated with reading handwritten physician orders.

In addition, there are many benefits anticipated to result from the use of electronic health (or medical) records (EHRs). One benefit is that EHRs will be accessible across providers and health systems, thus ensuring clear and complete communication on behalf of patients as they use various services. Online health records would have been helpful in the aftermath of Hurricane Katrina, for example, when large numbers of people were displaced with no records and no identification. In some cases, health records and vital statistics data were permanently lost.

One concern with EHRs is that information must be backed up regularly in the event of a system failure. Ensuring privacy of information remains another concern.

To date, fewer than 20% of hospitals or physician practices in the United States use EHRs. Purchasing and implementing the needed technology is costly, and many systems are reluctant to spend large amounts of money on implementing EHRs until consensus is reached about the standardization and interface of records across systems.

Disaster Preparedness

Disaster preparedness has been a part of health care protocols for many years, but it has taken a more prominent role in health care delivery since the World Trade Center events of September 11, 2001, and Hurricane Katrina in 2005. Disasters, always a part of everyday life, have been increasing due to the global instability, economic downturns, political upheavals and collapse of government structures, violence, civil conflicts, famine, and mass population displacements seen in the late 20th and early 21st centuries. The escalating nature and scope of disasters and their growing complexity provide challenges to health care institutions and health care workers responsible for disaster planning. Disasters are sudden, catastrophic events that can result in great damage, loss, injury, and death. They can be grouped into two types: unintentional and intentional.

Unintentional Disasters

Unintentional disasters are those that occur predominantly as a result of natural events. Natural disasters usually occur suddenly and are often uncontrollable, however, they frequently cluster in a certain time period or geographic location and, therefore, are somewhat predictable. In the United States and other developed countries, most natural disasters tend to cause extensive damage and social disruption with comparatively little loss of life. Unintentional disasters include such events as tsunamis, floods, typhoons, earthquakes, and epidemics. The response to unintentional disasters may be local or worldwide depending on the magnitude of the event. The most frequent natural or unintentional disasters experienced in the United States are floods, earthquakes, hurricanes, tornados, and fires.

Intentional Disasters

Intentional disasters are those that occur as the result of human purpose; that is, they are man-made or the result of human intervention and include such events as terrorism, bioterrorism, chemical releases, nuclear accidents, and explosions directly associated with human action. They can be caused by deliberate malicious activities or when industrial facilities are disrupted by natural disasters. Intentional disasters share many of the characteristics of natural ones but are typically less predictable.

Role of Health Care Professionals

Health care workers are on the front lines when a disaster occurs, therefore, nurses and other health care personnel need to have a basic understanding of disaster preparedness. All nurses need to know how to keep themselves and their patients and families safe during any disaster event.

Disaster nursing differs from emergency nursing in several ways. Emergency nursing usually involves nursing care for patients with acute injuries or life-threatening illnesses and is usually administered in an emergency department or on a trauma unit. Disaster nursing involves providing care in response to natural and man-made events that affect entire communities.

The widespread injury and disruption associated with disasters can pose difficult problems for health care providers, including the triage of mass casualties, disruption of infrastructure (e.g., loss of power and fresh water), and the need to deal with the mental anguish associated with uncertainty and the loss of loved ones. The outcome of a disaster is influenced by many factors, including population location and density, timing of the event, and community preparedness (e.g., emergency response infrastructure). Similarly, recovery after a disaster is influenced by resources (e.g., savings, insurance, and relief aid), pre-existing conditions (e.g., season of the year, local infrastructure, etc.), experience, and access to information. In almost all cases, disasters are associated with mental and physical stress (both during and after the event) that can increase morbidity and mortality over and above that caused directly by the event itself (Veenema, 2007).

Disaster Plans

Most hospitals and other health care facilities have disaster plans in place. These plans should address four phases: preparedness, identification, response, and recovery. All health care providers should be aware of the plans drawn up by their institution and know their role should a disaster occur. States and cities have implemented disaster preparedness procedures to coordinate government and health system effectiveness.

Preparedness. Developing, testing, and maintaining a plan for handling unexpected events will yield a fast and effective response should a disaster occur. Preparedness includes identifying key emergency personnel (e.g., law enforcement, health care and fire personnel, and school administrators), identifying areas of vulnerability (e.g., events/ facilities that have a large number of people present, food and water systems, etc.), developing a comprehensive security plan and disaster response plan, and conducting and maintaining the training of responders. In this stage, the community's and the health care institution's ability to respond is assessed.

Identification. A basic element for minimizing loss during a disaster is rapid identification that an event has occurred. That translates into knowing when something unusual is occurring within the local community, recognizing it, and reporting it to the appropriate authorities.

Response. While a disaster is unfolding and until control of the event has been established, the two-way communication of information

becomes paramount. Questions, concerns, and facts should be collected and channeled to appropriate agencies while information
from those agencies is disseminated to responders and to the public.
Volunteers and first responders, such as police, fire, and health care
personnel, are mobilized to assess the extent of the disaster and to
respond.

Recovery. Recovery from a disaster will be a long process and will
require local personnel and agencies that know and understand the
community and how it functions. Impacted areas will require follow-
up interaction, education, and assistance to minimize short-term and
long-term consequences. Because this is a long-term process, the approach will require an evaluation of the disaster response team and
the development of a new or revised plan of work for recovery.

ACCESS TO HEALTH CARE INFORMATION

Access to information on health care providers and health conditions
is increasingly available to consumers through a variety of sources. For
example, Medicare provides public access to information related to
quality of care in hospitals, skilled nursing facilities, and home health
agencies via the Internet. Many states are creating publicly accessible
databases that enable health care consumers to examine quality outcome data about providers and hospitals. The Agency for Healthcare
Research and Quality (AHRQ) offers consumers an extensive Web
site with information about safety in general and standards of care for
specific conditions (2008).

The Internet has generated an explosion of information that consumers can access. Hospitals, particularly academic medical centers,
often have extensive Web sites that offer information to patients about
specific conditions and how they are managed. U.S. organizations
that advocate on behalf of the prevention and treatment of specific
diseases and conditions, such as the American Cancer Society and
the American Heart Association, offer extensive information about
these conditions, and it is increasingly common for patients to approach health care providers with information about their conditions.

Information shared by patients should be regarded with respect, and patients need to be viewed as collaborators in their own care. That does not mean that all health information is of high quality; therefore, all health professionals, including nurses, need to help patients understand which information is useful and why.

ALTERNATIVE HEALTH PRACTICES

Patients and families in the United States make extensive use of health practices that are outside the health care system, although increasingly, health care institutions are incorporating some of these strategies. These therapies often are referred to as complementary and alternative medicine.

According to a national survey conducted by the CDC's National Center for Health Statistics (2004), 36% of U.S. adults use some form of complementary therapy within a given year. When prayer is included, the number rises to 62%. The 10 most common modalities include prayer for own health (43%); prayer for health of another (24%); natural products including herbs, **botanicals,** and enzymes (19%); deep breathing exercises (12%); group prayer for own health (10%); meditation (8%); chiropractic (8%); yoga (5%); massage (5%); and diet therapies (4%).

Many prestigious medical centers have sought to integrate these modalities into conventional care. For example, Memorial Sloan-Kettering Cancer Center established its Integrative Medicine Service in 1999 to offer patients and their families a holistic approach to care that combines **alternative therapies** with mainstream cancer care. The National Institutes of Health (NIH) also has a national center for complementary and alternative medicine that has been operating since 1999.

SUMMARY

While it is impossible to provide an exhaustive description of the U.S. health care system within the scope of a single article or chapter, this chapter is an attempt to offer a broad overview of issues that shape the way individual patients access health care services. There is much that is good about the U.S. health care system. Innovation in **biomedical research,** delivery of services, and health professions education has contributed to a high quality of life in the United States. Still, challenges associated with access to care and the financing of health care, as well as guarantees of safe, high-quality care, remain to be solved.

REFERENCES

Agency for Healthcare Research and Quality. (2008). *AHRQ Annual Highlights, 2007.* Retrieved October 15, 2008, from http://www.ahrq.gov/about/highlt07.htm

Berwick, D. M., Calkins, D. R., McCannon, C. J., & Hackbarth, A. D. (2006). The 100,000 lives campaign: Setting a goal and a deadline for improving health care quality. *Journal of the American Medical Association, 295*(3), 324–327.

Bureau of Labor Statistics. (2008). *Occupational employment statistics. List of SOC occupations. U.S. Department of Labor Bureau of Labor Statistics.* Retrieved October 25, 2008, from http://www.bls.gov/oes/current/oes_stru.htm#29-0000

Centers for Disease Control and Prevention. (2008a). *About CDC.* Retrieved October 15, 2008, from http://www.cdc.gov/about/

Centers for Disease Control and Prevention. (2008b). *Chronic disease overview.* Retrieved January 29, 2009, from http://www.cdc.gov/NCCdphp/overview.htm

Centers for Disease Control and Prevention. (2008c). *Overweight and obesity.* Retrieved October 15, 2008, from http://cdc.gov/nccdphp/dnpa/obesity/

Centers for Medicare and Medicaid Services. (2008). Center for Medicaid and State Operations. Letter of July 31, 2008. Retrieved October 15, 2008, from http://www.cms.hhs.gov/SMDL/downloads/SMD073108.pdf

Chua, K.-P. (2006). *Overview of the U.S. Health Care System. American Medical Student Association.* Retrieved October 12, 2008, from http://www.amsa.org/uhc/HealthcareSystemOverview.pdf

Corporate Research Group. (2008). *Best practices of on-site employee health clinics: Strategies for success.* New Rochelle, NY: Corporate Research Group.

Health Care Without Harm. (2008). *About us.* Retrieved October 15, 2008, from http://www.noharm.org/us/aboutUs/missionGoals

Hospicenet. (2008). *Hospice.* Retrieved October 15, 2008, from http://www.hospicenet.org/index.html

Institute for Healthcare Improvement. (2008). *Protecting 5,000,000 lives.* Retrieved October 15, 2008, from http://www.ihi.org/IHI/Programs/Campaign/

Institute of Medicine. (1994). *Defining primary care: An interim report.* Washington, DC: National Academies Press.

Institute of Medicine. (1999). *To err is human: Building a safer health system.* Washington, DC: National Academies Press.

The Joint Commission. (2008). *Home care.* Retrieved October 15, 2008, from http://www.jointcommission.org/AccreditationPrograms/HomeCare

The Leapfrog Group. (2008). *The Leapfrog Group fact sheet.* Retrieved October 15, 2008, from http://www.leapfroggroup.org/about_us/leapfrog-factsheet

Medicare. (2008a). *Long term care.* Retrieved October 15, 2008, from http://www.medicare.gov/longtermcare/static/home.asp

Medicare. (2008b). *Medicare.* Retrieved October 29, 2008, from http://www.medicare.gov/

National Center for Health Statistics. (2004). *More than one-third of U.S. adults use complementary and alternative medicine.* Retrieved January 18, 2009, from http://www.cdc.gov/nchs/pressroom/04news/adultsmedicine/htm

Supportive Care Coalition, (2008). *About the coalition.* Retrieved October 15, 2008, from http://www.supportivecarecoalition.org/AboutCoalition/mission_statement.htm

Urgent Care Association of America. (2008). *About urgent care.* Retrieved October 15, 2008, from http://www.ucaoa.org/home_abouturgentcare.php

Veenema, T. G. (Ed.). (2007). *Disaster nursing and emergency preparedness for chemical, biological and radiological terrorism and other hazards* (2nd ed.). New York: Springer Publishing.

Zhan, C., & Miller, M. E. (2003). Excess length of stay, charges, and mortality attributable to medical injuries during hospitalization. *Journal of the American Medical Association, 290*(14), 1868–1874.

7

Nursing Practice in the United States

WINIFRED Y. CARSON-SMITH
BARBARA L. NICHOLS

In This Chapter

Diversity in Health Care

Factors Influencing the Registered Nurse's Role in the U.S. Health Care System

Nursing Across the Life Span

Nursing Process

Summary

Keywords

Accreditation: Type of quality assurance process under which services and operations of an institution or program are evaluated by an external body to determine if applicable standards are met. Should standards be met, accredited status is granted by the external body.

Advanced practice nurses (APNs): Registered nurses who are educated at the master's level; have advanced theory and clinical education, knowledge, skills, and scope of practice; and can practice as independent practitioners. Includes nurse practitioners, clinical nurse specialists, certified nurse anesthetists, and certified nurse midwives.

Certification: Reflects achievement beyond the basic level of nursing and possession of expert knowledge in a particular area of practice.

The Joint Commission: Independent, nonprofit organization that evaluates and accredits more than 15,000 health care organizations and programs in the United States; the nation's predominant standards-setting and accrediting body in health care.

Nurse Practice Act: Group of laws governing nursing practice.

Nursing process: A step-by-step, problem-solving approach that includes assessment, analysis or diagnosis, planning, implementation, and evaluation.

Scope of practice: Refers to what a professional is legally authorized to do.

Specialty certification: Validation of competence, recognition of excellence, or legal recognition in a specialty area of practice.

NURSING IN THE UNITED STATES

The level of autonomy associated with nursing practice in the United States is likely to be different from that to which many foreign-educated nurses are accustomed. This chapter defines and describes nursing practice in the United States, the laws that govern professional practice, and the standards of practice, education, and ethical conduct that nurses are expected to meet. The authority to practice nursing is defined and governed by law, and entry into the profession is regulated at the state level.

Nurses across the world have much in common in their professional commitment to providing safe, high-quality care and improving the health of individuals, families, and communities. In fact, your ability to enter the United States to work as a nurse depends in part on demonstrating that your nursing education is comparable to the level of education required of U.S. nurses. At the same time, nursing in every country has its own history, traditions, and legal framework for defining the profession.

LAWS AND REGULATIONS THAT GOVERN NURSING PRACTICE

In order to understand the laws and regulations that govern nursing practice, it is helpful to know a little bit about the system of government in the United States. Both federal and state governments are composed of three equal branches: legislative, executive, and judicial. Under the 10th Amendment to the U.S. Constitution, all powers not granted to the federal government are reserved for the states and the people. All state governments are modeled after the federal government.

Legislative Branch of Government

The legislative branch of government has the authority to make laws, that is, it discusses and passes laws, which are sometimes referred to as statutes or legislation. At the federal level, the legislative branch is the U.S. Congress, which includes the U.S. Senate and the U.S. House of Representatives. Each state also has its own legislature, including a Senate and a House of Representatives, the members of which are elected by voters in local districts around the state.

Executive Branch of Government

While the legislative branch makes the laws, the executive branch of government is responsible for implementing and enforcing the laws written by Congress. In the federal government, the head of the executive branch is the president of the United States. In state government, the executive branch is headed by the state governor. The president and the state governors are elected officials.

At both the federal and state levels, the executive branch also includes a number of governmental agencies. The head officials of federal governmental agencies are appointed by the president. The head officials of the state governmental agencies are appointed by the governor. In almost all cases, the heads of state agencies, such as those related to health, are appointed, but this may differ from state to state.

Governmental Agencies

Governmental agencies are responsible for carrying out the laws enacted by the legislative branch on a day-to-day basis. In order to do this, the agencies often have to define how to carry out those laws. This is generally done by issuing regulations (sometimes referred to as rules).

For example, in 1994, California's state legislature passed a law (Assembly Bill 394) requiring hospitals to determine their nurse staffing levels based on ratios; that is, by limiting the numbers of patients that a licensed nurse could provide care for at any one time.

However, the law did not specify the actual number of patients per nurse, or whether a certain percentage of the nurses had to be registered nurses (RNs) as opposed to licensed vocational nurses (LVNs). The job of filling in these details was left up to a state health agency (then known as the California Department of Health Services), which did so by issuing regulations on nurse-to-patient ratios.

Judicial Branch of Government

The third branch of government is the judicial branch—the court system. At the federal level, this is the Supreme Court, which is the highest court in the United States. Whereas the executive and legislative branches of the federal government are elected by the people, members of the judicial branch are appointed by the president and confirmed by the U.S. Senate. State judicial branches are usually led by the state supreme court. Local judges may be appointed or elected.

The judicial branch of government interprets the law and acts as a competent administrator to ensure compliance with the laws crafted by the legislative branch of government. Among other responsibilities, the courts are often called upon to decide on disputes about laws that have been passed by the legislatures, or regulations that have been issued by government agencies. The judiciary also is where malpractice and professional misconduct cases and end-of-life questions are decided.

TITLES OF PRACTITIONERS

Each state has a group of laws governing nursing practice. These laws are usually referred to collectively as the state's **Nurse Practice Act.** The laws generally include requirements for eligibility for nursing licensure, standards for nursing education programs, and a description of the **scope of practice** of RNs, licensed practical nurses (LPNs), and **advanced practice nurses** (such as nurse practitioners). The scope of practice refers to what a professional is legally authorized to do.

The Nurse Practice Act also establishes which state agency is responsible for regulating nursing practice. This differs from state to state. In California, the state agency responsible for licensing and regulating the health professions is the Department of Consumer Affairs. In New York, the responsible agency is a division of the State Education Department. In Washington State, the agency is the Nursing Care Quality Assurance Commission and is part of the state Department of Public Health.

In addition to identifying requirements for licensure, these laws also identify the titles and define the scopes of practice of those functioning within the law. The titles most commonly identified in the Nurse Practice Acts are registered nurse, advanced practice nurse, licensed practical nurse, licensed vocational nurse, nursing assistant, and nursing student. These titles are described throughout this chapter.

RESPONSIBILITIES OF STATE BOARDS OF NURSING

In each state, standards for most of the health professions, including nursing, are determined and enforced by a board—a group of individuals who have been appointed to help govern the practice of a profession in that state. For nursing, that board is known in almost all states as the Board of Nursing. Some states may use slightly different terminology. For example, in Indiana, the board is officially known as the Indiana State Board for Nursing Professional Licensing Agency, but in Massachusetts, it is called the Massachusetts Board of Registration in Nursing. However, each is considered the Board of Nursing for that state.

In most states, both RNs and LPNs (known in California and Texas as licensed vocational nurses, or LVNs) are regulated by a single board. In four states, there are separate boards for RNs and LPNs/LVNs. So, for example, California has a Board of Registered Nursing and a Board of Vocational Nurse and Psychiatric Technician Examiners.

Board of Nursing Membership

Members of the Board of Nursing are private individuals, that is, they are not full-time government employees. In almost every state, the members of the Board are appointed to serve for a specific term of office, for example, for 4 years. Each state's Nurse Practice Act generally sets out how many Board of Nursing members must be RNs and/or LPNs. This is in keeping with the idea of professional self-regulation—the idea being that nurses are the experts on nursing practice, education, standards of practice, and ethical conduct. The state Nurse Practice Act may specify that a certain number of Board members must meet specific additional qualifications; for example, some must be nurse educators and one or more must be a staff nurse, a nurse administrator, or an advanced practice nurse.

The traditional approach of having health licensing boards composed solely of members of the profession has been at least somewhat modified in most states. Because the primary purpose of the Boards is to protect the public, some critics questioned whether professional licensing boards that are dominated by members of the profession might be too protective of their colleagues. For the most part, examples supporting these concerns were drawn from other professional licensing boards, such as Boards of Medicine, not Boards of Nursing. Thus, most states also include a specified number of public members, that is, members who are not nurses or other health professionals.

Board Role in Nursing Practice and Education

The Board of Nursing plays an important role in nursing practice and education. It adopts or recommends regulations implementing the Nurse Practice Act, which may include providing important details such as specific requirements for nursing curricula, specifics of continuing education requirements (if any), and often details of the scope of practice of RNs and LPNs.

The Board also may approve schools of nursing in that state. In addition, the Board establishes the standards for nursing education programs preparing for nursing licensure. These standards are designed to ensure that graduates have the necessary education to safely and competently practice nursing. The Board of Nursing also conducts an in-person review of the schools to make sure that their curriculum, including clinical placement and experiences, meet the state requirements. Those schools that do meet the requirements are identified as having State Board approval. Graduates of an unapproved school would not be eligible for licensure in that state.

Board Role in Professional Discipline

Another important function of the Board of Nursing is to carry out the state's system of professional discipline. If a nurse is accused of incompetence or unsafe practice, for example, the Board will determine whether that nurse has violated expected standards of professional performance. It will then decide what kind of disciplinary action the nurse will face, which can include revoking or suspending the nurse's license to practice. In assessing a nurse's performance, the Board will rely on standards contained in the Nurse Practice Act and in state regulations. The Board also may look to other sources of professional standards of practice and the *Code of Ethics for Nurses.*

Every nurse should know what is included in his or her state's Nurse Practice Act and in Board of Nursing regulations. In many states, a booklet containing these documents is provided by the Board to newly licensed nurses. This information generally is available on the Internet by going to the Web site of the state Board of Nursing, where you can access the Nurse Practice Act for that state. For example, the Nurse Practice Act for New York State may be accessed at http://www.op.nysed.gov/nurse.htm, for California at http://www.rn.ca.gov/pdfs/regulations/npr-b-03.pdf, and for New Jersey at http://www.state.nj.us/lps/ca/nursing/nurselaws.pdf. Nursing practice in New York State, for example, is defined by State Education Law, Article 139 (the Nurse Practice Act), which states:

> The practice of the profession of nursing as a registered professional nurse is defined as diagnosing and treating human responses to actual or potential health problems through such services as casefinding, health teaching, health counseling, and provision of care supportive to or restorative of life and well-being, and executing medical regimens prescribed by a licensed physician, dentist or other licensed health care provider legally authorized under this title and in accordance with the commissioner's regulations.

This definition authorizes RNs to execute medical orders from certain authorized health care providers. RNs also may function independently in providing nursing care related to casefinding, health teaching, health counseling, and provision of care supportive to or restorative of life and well-being.

PROFESSIONAL AUTONOMY AND INDEPENDENT ACCOUNTABILITY

Professional Autonomy

In the United States, nursing places great emphasis on having the authority to determine the standards of practice, education, and ethical conduct that members of the profession are expected to meet. The concept of professional autonomy and self-regulation means that the profession takes responsibility for setting its own standards. The nursing profession in the United States does this in various steps.

For example, the American Nurses Association (ANA) has adopted the following definition of nursing: "Nursing is the protection, promotion and optimization of health and abilities, prevention of illness and injury, alleviation of suffering through the diagnosis and treatment of human response, and advocacy in the care of individuals, families, communities, and populations" (ANA, 2003, p. 6).

ANA also develops and publishes standards of nursing practice that provide guidelines for nursing performance. These standards represent the definition or benchmark of what it means to provide competent care. By law, the RN is required to provide care in accordance with what other reasonable nurses would do in the same or similar circumstances. In other words, provision of care consistent with established standards is expected. Thus, the standards represent national measures of professional practice.

As defined by the ANA, standards of nursing practice consist of three components:

1. Professional Standards of Care—define diagnostic, intervention, and evaluation competencies.

2. Professional Performance Standards—identify role functions in direct care, consultation, and quality assurance.
3. Specialty Practice Guidelines—identify protocols of care for specific populations.

ANA has developed and published standards for clinical nursing practice and specialty practice, including public health nursing. Copies of

Exhibit 7.1

Current Scope and Standards of Practice as Provided by the American Nurses Association

Scope and Standards of Hospice and Palliative Nursing Practice

Genetics/Genomics Nursing: Scope and Standards of Practice

Scope and Standards of Neuroscience Nursing Practice

Scope and Standards of Psychiatric-Mental Health Nursing Practice

Scope and Standards of Addictions Nursing Practice

Intellectual And Developmental Disabilities Nursing: Scope and Standards of Practice

HIV/AIDS Nursing: Scope and Standards of Practice

Scope and Standards of Diabetes Nursing Practice

Scope and Standards of Vascular Nursing Practice

Scope and Standards of Gerontological Nursing Practice

Plastic Surgery Nursing: Scope and Standards of Practice

Scope and Standards of Pediatric Nursing Practice

School Nursing: Scope and Standards of Practice

Neonatal Nursing: Scope and Standards of Practice

Scope and Standards of Nursing Informatics Practice

Legal Nurse Consulting: Scope and Standards of Practice

Scope and Standards of Practice of Nursing Professional Development

Nursing: Scope and Standards of Practice

Radiology Nursing: Scope and Standards of Practice

Pain Management Nursing: Scope and Standards of Practice

Scope and Standards for Nursing Administrators

Public Health Nursing: Scope and Standards of Practice

Scope and Standards of Home Health Nursing Practice

Faith Community Nursing: Scope and Standards of Practice

Note: All are available for purchase through the ANA Web site: http://nursingworld.org.

the standards can be ordered from the ANA at http://nursingworld. org/books/. A listing is shown in Exhibit 7.1.

ANA and other nursing organizations play a role in setting the standards for the profession:

- ANA adopted and periodically updates *Nursing: Scopes and Standards of Practice* (ANA, 2004), which describes the parameters of professional nursing and explains the expected functions and responsibilities of professional nurses.
- Nursing specialty organizations, often in collaboration with ANA, adopt and update scope and standards statements for nurses practicing within their specialties.
- The American Nurses Credentialing Center (ANCC) and many specialty nursing **certification** boards certify nurses who demonstrate proficiency or expertise in a large number of specialty areas and nursing roles. Certification is based on professional standards, such as the scope and standards statements.
- Nursing education programs are accredited through certifying bodies, such as the Certification Commission for Nursing Education (CCNE) and the National League for Nursing Accrediting Commission (NLNAC), based on standards developed and adopted by nurse educators and education leaders.
- ANA adopted and periodically revises the *Code of Ethics for Nurses* (ANA, 2001) to provide guidance for ethical conduct and decision making and to describe the nursing profession's obligation to society.

Independent Accountability

Professional accountability—being responsible for your actions and for the outcomes of these actions—is a hallmark of nursing practice. As independently licensed professionals, nurses are accountable for their own actions. This does not mean, however, that they practice in isolation.

Dependent Nursing Functions

Many nursing functions are *dependent* on other professionals. For example, nurses cannot administer medications without an order from a physician or another health care professional who is authorized to write prescriptions, such as a nurse practitioner. However, even when implementing physician or nurse practitioner orders, nurses are accountable for exercising independent judgment. For example, if a nurse receives a medication order that is erroneous or dangerous (such as an inappropriately high dosage, or an order for a medication to which the patient has a known allergy), the nurse has a responsibility to question the order and even to refuse to administer it and to notify the appropriate supervisor.

Interdependent Nursing Functions

Some other nursing functions are considered *interdependent;* that is, they emphasize collaboration with other professionals. Nursing's interdependent role concerns the activities and functions in which nurses engage that are partially or totally dependent on the functions of other providers of health care. It also includes those activities of the nurse on which other health care professionals depend for accomplishing their own activities.

Examples of nurses' interdependent role function include promoting continuity of care and coordinating care. Even when nurses engage in interdependent nursing functions, they are still accountable for their own actions.

Independent Nursing Functions

Other nursing functions are *independent.* Nursing's independent role concerns the role functions and responsibilities for which only nurses are held accountable. They include the activities of assessment, decision making, intervention, and follow-up that define the **nursing process.**

Registered nurses assess patients in order to determine judgment in providing care. They also assess patients to determine patient needs and the most effective patient care interventions. The continued development of advanced practice roles, for example, has helped to further define the independent and autonomous features of nursing practice in the United States.

NURSING SPECIALIZATION AND CERTIFICATION

In the United States, nursing, unlike many other professions, has no single authoritative source for recognizing specialties. "Nursing specialties originate and are recognized in numerous and various ways, e.g., through educational programs, state certification or 'second licensing' programs, national certification programs, specialty organizations and councils, and job descriptions" (Styles, Schumann, Bickford, & White, 2008, p. 115).

Nursing Specialization

Specialization in nursing is dynamic and rapidly changing. Specialties are emerging from functional roles such as administration and teaching, and levels of patient acuity such as emergency care, critical care, chronic illness, or primary care. For example, nurses use their specialized knowledge and skills to provide care in operating rooms as surgical nurses, working as circulating or scrub nurses. They may work as gerontological nurses, providing care to the growing U.S. elderly population, or they may work as community health nurses, assisting patients who require on-going care in their homes and other community-based settings. Still other nurses may specialize in nursing education, which requires higher education, such as a master's or doctoral degree. These nurses teach nursing and health care in schools of nursing.

Specialty Certification

In order to understand the standards that govern specialty nurse certification, it is helpful to generally explain the role of certification in the nursing profession. Like specialization, the role of certification is multifaceted and complex. While licensure by a State Board of Nursing provides for entry into nursing practice, certification by a private **specialty certification** body reflects achievement beyond the basic level of nursing.

Given the importance of the credentialing organizations in the nurse specialty certification process, they, too, are subject to state regulations. And, as such, professional standards developed by national nursing organizations have been used to assist State Boards of Nursing in evaluating nurse credentialing organizations.

Certification can be used for validation of competence, recognition of competency, recognition of excellence, or legal recognition in a specialty area of practice. It can be mandatory, academic, or professional.

Development of Specialty Certification

The American Board of Nursing Specialties (ABNS, 2000) defines *certification* "as the formal recognition of the specialized knowledge, skills and experience demonstrated by the achievement of standards identified by a nursing specialty to promote optimal health outcomes." The ANA established its Certification Program in 1973 to provide tangible recognition of professional achievement in a defined functional or clinical area of nursing. In 1975, ANA issued its first specialty certification.

That same year, ANA's Division on Maternal and Child Health Nursing Practice and the Nurses Association of the American College of Obstetricians and Gynecologists initiated a joint certification program in maternal, gynecological, and neonatal nursing. Subsequently, in 1991, the ANCC became its own corporation and a subsidiary of ANA.

Types of Specialty Certification

Certification is reserved for those nurses who have met requirements for clinical or functional practice in a specialized field. Specialty certification validates a nurse's knowledge, skills, and abilities in a specialty area of practice. There are two types of certification: generalist level and advanced practice. Each has different eligibility requirements (ANCC, 2009).

Generalist level certification requires the nurse to be licensed as an RN, to have practiced as an RN for a specified amount of time, to have the prescribed number of hours of practice in the specialty area, and to have a prescribed number of hours of continuing education in the specialty area. Nurses who hold generalist level certification cannot practice as independent practitioners nor can they bill for, or be reimbursed for, their services.

Advanced practice certification is reserved for those nurses who hold a master's degree and were educated as advanced practice nurses (nurse practitioners, clinical nurse specialists, nurse midwives, or nurse anesthetists) or are engaged in an advanced level of nursing practice in a nursing specialty (e.g., public health nurse–advanced).

Process of Specialty Certification

A nurse seeking professional certification must meet education, practice, and experience requirements and successfully complete a comprehensive national examination that assesses the nurse's knowledge and skills in the specialty. The certification process provides assurance to the public that the nurse has met established standards and the level of competence in the specialty that is required for certification.

Once the certification is earned it must be renewed on a schedule required by the certifying agency. Recertification is required to maintain the certification and to demonstrate continued competency in the specialty.

There are 31 nursing specialty certifications that are accepted by virtually every State Board of Nursing. However, most specialty certifications are offered by the following accrediting entities:

- American Nurses Credentialing Center
- American Academy of Nurse Practitioners Certification Program
- American Midwifery Certification Board
- National Board on Certification and Recertification of Nurse Anesthetists
- National Certification Corporation for the Obstetric, Gynecological, and Neonatal Specialties
- Pediatric Nursing Certification
- American Association of Critical Care Nurses Certification Corporation

A more comprehensive list of nursing specialty organizations and their Web addresses may be found in chapter 11, Table 11.3.

Accreditation of Certification Agencies

The National Commission on Certifying Agencies (NCCA) was created in 1987 to ensure the health, welfare, and safety of the public through the **accreditation** of a variety of certification programs/organizations that determine professional competence. Certification programs that receive NCCA accreditation demonstrate compliance with the NCCA's *Standards for the Accreditation of Certification Programs,* which were the first standards for professional certification programs developed by the industry (NCCA, 2009).

NCCA uses a peer-review process to establish accreditation standards, evaluate compliance with the standards, and to recognize organizations or programs that demonstrate compliance. Certification organizations can submit their programs for NCCA review and accreditation (NCCA, 2009).

In response to a need to be more formally organized as a national peer review program for nursing certification, the ANCC and more than a dozen certification boards joined the ABNS. The Accreditation Council of ABNS is the only accrediting body specifically for nursing certification.

The Accreditation Council, an autonomous body responsible for decisions regarding accreditation of specialty nursing certifications, provides a process for accrediting nursing certification examinations for both member and nonmember organizations. This is a peer-review mechanism that allows nursing certification organizations to obtain accreditation by demonstrating compliance with established ABNS Accreditation Council standards (ABNS, 2000).

ADVANCED PRACTICE NURSING

Advanced practice nurses (APNs) are registered nurses who are educated at the master's level and have advanced theory and clinical education, knowledge, skills, and scope of practice. They can practice as independent practitioners and can be directly reimbursed by health insurance plans for the care they provide. Every state has different licensing and certification requirements for advanced practice nurses.

The term *advanced practice nurse* is actually a blanket term used to describe four separate, graduate-level professions within the nursing profession as a whole: nurse practitioners, certified registered nurse anesthetists, clinical nurse specialists, and certified nurse midwives.

Nurse practitioners (NPs) provide basic care focused on a specific population or health need, with the ability to write prescriptions. Family nurse practitioners and pediatric nurse practitioners are two examples.

Certified registered nurse anesthetists (CRNAs) administer anesthesia for all types of surgery and provide clinical support services outside of the operating room. CRNAs practice in every setting in which anesthesia is delivered, including such areas as traditional hospital surgical suites, obstetrical delivery rooms, physicians' offices, and ambulatory surgical centers.

The *clinical nurse specialist* (CNS) provides specialized care (clinical practice, teaching, research, consulting, and management) for certain types of diseases (such as diabetes or cardiovascular disease), in certain medical environments (such as operating room, emergency room, or critical care), for specific patient populations (such as geriatric or neonatal patients), or for specialized procedures (such as surgical).

Certified nurse midwives (CNMs) provide prenatal care, deliver babies, and provide postpartum care to normal healthy women. In addition, CNMs provide family planning, birth control counseling, and normal gynecological services such as physical and breast exams, pap smears, and preventive health screening. In most states, CNMs may prescribe medications.

Advanced Practice Specialty Certification

With the creation of APN roles, boards of nursing and the profession sought to legitimize the positions. In response to this need, nurse credentialing organizations began to study how to address competency in advanced practice nursing. The current system for recognizing APNs through certification was established and is operated by professional nursing specialty organizations.

Boards of Nursing usually require APNs to provide evidence of specialty certification by a nursing organization. States that also issue an advanced practice license (in addition to the RN license) have both education and certification requirements. These standards enforce uniformity to ensure that all nurses with the specialty certification have been educated as APNs and have competence in their specialty at the advanced practice nursing level.

Regulation of Advanced Practice Nurses

Education, accreditation, and certification are necessary components of an overall approach to preparing APNs for practice. Currently, there is no uniform model of regulation of APNs across the states. Each state independently determines the APN legal scope of practice, the roles that are recognized, the criteria for entry into advanced practice, and the certification examinations accepted for entry-level competence assessment (National Council of State Boards of Nursing, 2008).

While the requirements are not consistent across states, they do provide a mechanism for evaluating education and competence. Some states allow specialty certification in a limited number of areas. Other states include mechanisms for nurses to prove specialty competence, such as additional education, testing, or experience in the specialty as indicated by portfolio and other credentialing mechanisms. Certifications, like licenses, are time sensitive and must be renewed, usually every 4 or 5 years. One must have current certification for licensure as an APN.

Licensure Examination

Nursing organizations recently voted to change the regulatory mechanism for APNs so as to develop an examination akin to the NCLEX-RN. This examination will test advanced practice nursing core competencies to ensure a base level of advanced practice RN education.

When this examination is developed, the APN will be able to practice as a generalist but will have the option to retain, and have the Board of Nursing continue to certify the nurse in, an advanced practice nursing specialty. The specialty will be considered an addition, not the foundation of advanced practice nursing licensure.

REGULATION OF LICENSED PRACTICAL NURSES, NURSING STUDENTS, AND NURSING ASSISTANTS

Licensed Practical Nurses

Licensed practical nurses (LPNs) are supervised by and function under the delegated authority of the RN. Practical nurses provide care to patients that does not require the specialized skill, judgment, and knowledge of an RN. In addition, LPNs are not prepared for management or teaching positions.

The Nurse Practice Act defines requirements for eligibility for LPN licensure, standards for practical nursing education programs, and a description of the scope of practice. Licensed practical nurses, in their assistive role, work with RNs in all settings.

Regulation of Nursing Students

Nursing students are unregulated workers who are required to work under the supervision of a regulated member of a health profession and to perform the restricted activities that an RN or LPN is authorized to practice under the state law. Most states do not have a law that addresses the regulation of student nursing practice, although a few states do have regulations or advisory opinions on student nurse practice. U.S. graduate nurses (those who have graduated from their basic nursing education program) may practice for a limited amount of time until they pass the U.S. licensing examination.

Regulation of Nursing Assistants

Nursing assistants are unregulated workers who are required to work under the supervision of a regulated member of a health care profession and may only perform restricted activities that an RN or LPN is authorized to practice under state law. Nursing assistants are supervised by the RN and function in an assistive role under the delegated authority of the RN.

Nursing assistant training programs are conducted in private, for-profit schools, in vocational schools, and in employment settings as on-the-job training. Most states do not have a law that addresses the regulation of nursing assistants.

RELATIONSHIP OF NURSING TO OTHER HEALTH CARE PROVIDERS

The legislative process is designed to determine the nature and extent to which other health professions are able to provide care. Other licensed professions are granted scopes of practice, and while none of the scopes of the health professions is totally exclusive of others, the core or essence of any profession remains distinct. The numbers and types of health professions that are being regulated continue to expand. Originally, only nursing, medicine, and dentistry were regulated. Now, over 30 professions are regulated, including:

- Dentistry
- Occupational therapy
- Physical therapy
- Optometry
- Podiatry
- Audiology
- Dental technician
- Pharmacy
- Pharmacy technician
- Naturopathy
- Dietician and nutritionist

Each of these professions has its own scope of practice and rules related to practice. However, while there is a core for each profession, there are some procedures, standards, and practices that are common to various health professionals. The overlap is especially prominent between the scope of practice of nurse practitioners and medicine.

Medical professionals, the first licensed health profession, initially defined the scope of medicine to incorporate all health-related practices and procedures. While the licensed scope of practice of medicine remains the same today, technology and patient need has expanded the scopes of practice of other health care professions, such as nursing. In addition, new health care professions have been created that are specialized in nature and that have grown out of other licensed professions. This overlap creates confusion about what is perceived as each profession's specific scope of practice.

Technology is expanding to make the practice of nursing more efficient, to give nurses the ability to conduct complex procedures, and to address more complex nursing diagnoses. We will continue to see the scope of practice of nursing expand, along with an expansion of the tasks and roles of other health care professions.

OTHER AGENCIES THAT REGULATE HEALTH CARE

While the State Board of Nursing licenses RNs and LPNs and regulates their practice, there are several other agencies that regulate health care services and, therefore, have an important impact on nursing practice. For example, each state has a government agency that regulates hospitals, nursing homes, home health agencies, and other institutional providers. These agencies may be known by different names in different states, such as the Department of Health, the Department of Public Health, or the Department of Health Services, to name a few. Most states require hospitals to be licensed and to meet quality standards that are usually spelled out in state regulations.

The Joint Commission

Most hospitals undergo accreditation by **The Joint Commission** (formerly known as the Joint Commission on Accreditation of Healthcare Organizations, or JCAHO). The Joint Commission is a national, voluntary accrediting agency that issues a series of standards for patient care and operations. The Joint Commission has increasingly focused on safer patient care practices and decreasing the incidence of medical error.

Accreditation by The Joint Commission is considered a mark of quality. Hospitals that are accredited by The Joint Commission are deemed by the federal government to be in compliance with the conditions of participation in the Medicare and Medicaid programs. This provides an additional incentive for hospitals to seek accreditation by The Joint Commission—although not all hospitals choose to seek it. Some smaller and rural hospitals forego accreditation because of the expense involved.

PROFESSIONAL PRACTICE ISSUES

In addition to state nursing laws and regulations, there are other important sources of information on current nursing practice issues. Many State Boards of Nursing issue statements, memoranda, or advisories giving the Board's opinion on issues or problems that nurses have brought to their attention. One such issue is patient abandonment.

Patient Abandonment

Nurses and nursing organizations in many states have asked their State Board of Nursing for clarification regarding patient abandonment. Nurses have a responsibility to provide care for the patients assigned to them. Leaving a patient without appropriate care would be considered unethical and unprofessional conduct. But what should happen when a nurse is *mandated* (ordered) to stay and work beyond his/her scheduled shift? This is often referred to as *mandatory overtime,* and it has been a controversial practice in many hospitals.

Mandatory Overtime

Many nursing organizations have raised objections to using mandatory overtime as a routine practice to make up for low staffing levels, and many nurses have expressed concern about patient safety when they are required to work 16 or more hours in a row. Some have also expressed concern that unplanned overtime interferes with family or school obligations. As a result of these concerns and objections, several state legislatures have passed laws prohibiting mandatory overtime.

In many hospitals, however, nurses who questioned the practice of mandatory overtime were told that if they refused to stay and work beyond their assigned shifts, they would be reported to the Board of Nursing for patient abandonment. Some Boards of Nursing were asked to clarify whether or not a nurse who refused mandatory overtime could, in fact, be charged with patient abandonment.

State Board Response

The response of one Board, the New York State Board of Nursing, helps to illustrate the approach that State Boards of Nursing have taken to respond to issues of patient abandonment. The New York Board decided that if a nurse has not accepted the assignment to work beyond his or her regular shift, that refusal is generally not considered patient abandonment. Their decision reads, in part: "Abandonment results when the nurse-patient relationship is terminated without making reasonable arrangements with an appropriate person so that nursing care by others can be continued" (New York State Education Department, 2002).

The decision to charge a nurse with abandonment will depend on an examination of all of the circumstances surrounding a particular situation as assessed by State Education Department staff in consultation with members of the State Board of Nursing. Key questions to consider include:

- Did the nurse accept the patient assignment, thus establishing a nurse–patient relationship?
- Did the nurse provide reasonable notice when severing the nurse–patient relationship?
- Could reasonable arrangements have been made for continuation of nursing care by others when proper notification of patient assignment refusal was given?

An investigation of abandonment charges by the State Education Department would consider whether managerial or supervisory personnel made adequate provisions for competent staffing to ensure necessary patient care in routine situations. The Department and the nurse may obtain a copy of the nurse's written notice of patient assignment refusal in the event of such an investigation. The State Education Department views abandonment as a serious charge. It is, however, inappropriate for nurses to be threatened with charges of abandonment to coerce them to work additional hours or care for patients beyond their expertise.

Delegation

State Boards of Nursing and nursing professional organizations have worked to clarify issues surrounding another practice issue—delegation by nurses to other health care personnel. A variety of nursing personnel work together in patient care settings, for example, RNs, LPNs, and unlicensed personnel such as nursing assistants, nurses' aides, or patient care technicians. In the 1980s, many hospitals moved to all-RN staffing, but this is not a common staffing practice today. Instead, it is common for RNs to be assisted by LPNs and unlicensed personnel. RNs may assign some tasks and functions to LPNs; both RNs and LPNs may delegate tasks to unlicensed personnel. The use of the terms *assignment* and *delegation* may differ somewhat from state to state.

Joint Statement on Delegation

Nurses have posed many questions about what practices are safest, particularly in delegating tasks to unlicensed personnel. What are the limits on what an unlicensed person can be assigned? How much independent judgment should the nurse exercise in assigning tasks? How closely do unlicensed personnel need to be supervised?

In 2006, ANA and the National Council of State Boards of Nursing (NCSBN) adopted a joint statement on delegation. That statement noted:

- The RN assigns or delegates tasks based on the needs and condition of the patient, potential for harm, stability of the patient's condition, complexity of the task, predictability of the outcomes, abilities of the staff to whom the task is delegated, and the context of other patient needs.

■ All decisions related to delegation and assignment are based on the fundamental principles of protection of the health, safety, and welfare of the public.

■ The RN directs care and determines the appropriate utilization of any assistant involved in providing direct patient care.

■ The RN may delegate components of care but does not delegate the nursing process itself. The practice-pervasive functions of assessment, planning, evaluation, and nursing judgment cannot be delegated.

■ The decision of whether or not to delegate or assign is based upon the RN's judgment concerning the condition of the patient, the competence of all members of the nursing team, and the degree of supervision that will be required of the RN if a task is delegated.

■ The RN uses critical thinking and professional judgment when following the Five Rights of Delegation, to be sure that the delegation or assignment is:
  ■ The right task,
  ■ Under the right circumstances,
  ■ To the right person,
  ■ With the right decision and communication, and
  ■ Under the right supervision and evaluation.

■ Chief nursing officers are accountable for establishing systems to assess, monitor, verify, and communicate ongoing competence requirements in areas related to delegation. (American Nurses Association & National Council of State Boards of Nursing, 2006)

Legal Liability and Malpractice

As noted earlier, the judicial branch of government—the court system—also plays a role in health care services and nursing practice. The courts often are called upon to rule on whether or not specific federal and state laws are consistent with the U.S. or state constitutions. Courts also rule on accusations by the government of criminal wrong-doing by individuals.

Most relevant to nursing practice, however, is the role of the courts in resolving disputes between individuals. Courts often rule on disputes that arise over contracts—such as when one party to a contract claims that the other has breached the contract, or when one party claims that a contract should not be enforced.

Contract Disputes

In chapter 2 you read about contracts that nurses may be asked to sign with international recruitment agencies. If an agency or an employer believed that a nurse had violated his/her contract, they might choose to take that nurse to court to seek enforcement of the contract or to ask that the nurse be ordered to pay damages.

Conversely, a nurse might seek to take an agency or employer to court if the nurse believed that the contract was unfair and that he or she should be allowed to leave employment before the term of the contract. Also, a group of nurses might decide to sue their employer in order to collect the money they believe was owed to them if the contract promised a specific hourly wage but the employer paid a lower wage instead.

Negligence

Another law with which many U.S. health professionals are concerned is the law of negligence. Simply stated, *negligence* is when someone's failure to act with reasonable care results in harm (or damage) to another person. For example, if a driver carelessly fails to stop at a red light and, as a result, hits and injures a pedestrian, the injured pedestrian might decide to sue the driver in order to seek compensation for the injuries caused by the driver's negligence.

Malpractice

The term *malpractice* generally refers to negligence committed by a professional. Thus, *medical malpractice* generally refers to medical negligence. Physicians, nurses, and other health care professionals may be sued when a patient claims that he or she has been injured as the result of the physician or nurse acting negligently.

When a court examines a charge of malpractice against a nurse, it will consider whether the nurse failed to meet the applicable standard of care: Were the nurse's actions consistent with what a "reasonable" nurse would do in similar circumstances? What would nurses commonly or typically do in this situation?

For example, suppose Maria, a nurse on a medical–surgical unit, is preparing to administer morning medication for her patients. She has returned from a week's vacation and does not know any of her patients. One of her patients, Mr. Nguyen, is allergic to penicillin. Another patient, Mr. Garcia, has an order to receive penicillin. Maria is very busy that morning, and she does not check her patients' wristbands or ask them their names. Mr. Nguyen asks Maria what medications she is giving him, but she is in a hurry and just tells him, "These are the medications your doctor ordered for you." She mistakenly gives Mr. Nguyen the penicillin that was intended for Mr. Garcia. Mr. Nguyen suffers a severe allergic reaction.

If Mr. Nguyen decided to sue Maria, the court would want to consider whether Maria's actions violated the standard of care. Would nurses typically check to make sure they were administering the right medication to the right person? Would they provide information to the patient about his or her medications in response to a question by the patient? In answering these questions, the court might receive testimony from nursing experts, or examine what nursing textbooks say, or examine published statements by nursing organizations about standards of nursing practice. In fact, the court might do all of these things.

Malpractice Insurance

Many health professionals worry about the possibility of being sued. Anyone can make a mistake, even nurses and physicians who are usually very careful. In addition, health professionals often express concern about the possibility of being wrongfully sued. For these reasons, most physicians and many nurses carry malpractice insurance (also called *professional liability insurance*) to pay for legal representation and to help pay damages if they are found to be negligent. Although physicians' medical malpractice insurance rates are often very high, most nursing malpractice insurance policies are priced at less than $150 per year.

Most employers' malpractice policies cover negligence by employers under some circumstances. Thus, many nurses choose not to carry their own malpractice insurance. However, some experts argue that employers' policies do not provide sufficient protection to nurses and that nurses, because they are professionals in their own right, should carry their own individual policies.

Many health professionals believe that there are too many lawsuits in the United States and that one result of having too many lawsuits is to drive up health care costs. Some experts dispute these beliefs, but many physician and hospital groups have pushed for *tort reform*—reforms to the laws related to negligence and, especially, to medical malpractice that would limit the amounts the patient could sue for and receive in settlement. The reforms also would mandate arbitration as a first step.

CODE OF ETHICS

As autonomous professionals, nurses are expected to uphold the ethical principles of the profession. The *Code of Ethics for Nurses* (ANA, 2001) is both a guide for ethical nursing practice and a statement of the profession's obligation to the public we serve. While nursing has always emphasized the importance of ethical behavior, the profession's first Code of Ethics was adopted by ANA in 1953. The Code has gone through several revisions and updates since then in order to remain relevant to current practice. The most recent revision of the Code was adopted in 2001 and consists of nine provisions:

1. The nurse, in all professional relationships, practices with compassion and respect for the inherent dignity, worth, and uniqueness of every individual, unrestricted by considerations

of social or economic status, personal attributes, or the nature of health problems.

2. The nurse's primary commitment is to the patient, whether an individual, family, group, or community.
3. The nurse promotes, advocates for, and strives to protect the health, safety, and rights of the patient.
4. The nurse is responsible and accountable for individual nursing practice and determines the appropriate delegation of tasks consistent with the nurse's obligation to provide optimum patient care.
5. The nurse owes the same duties to self as to others, including the responsibility to preserve integrity and safety, to maintain competence, and to continue personal professional growth.
6. The nurse participates in establishing, maintaining, and improving health care environments and conditions of employment conducive to the provision of quality health care and consistent with the values of the profession through individual and collective action.
7. The nurse participates in the advancement of the profession though contributions to practice, education, administration, and knowledge development.
8. The nurse collaborates with other health care professionals and the public in promoting community, national, and international efforts to meet health needs.
9. The profession of nursing, as represented by associations and their members, is responsible for articulating nursing values, for maintaining the integrity of the profession and its practice, and for shaping social policy. (ANA, 2001)

New Elements of the Code of Ethics

The Code of Ethic's emphasis on the nurse's primary duty to the patient (Provision 2) is consistent with previous versions of the Code. However, the current version of the Code includes some points that previously had not been emphasized. For example, Provision 4 notes the importance of appropriate delegation (an issue discussed previously in this chapter). Provision 5 emphasizes that "The nurse owes the same duties to self as to others." To many people, this statement seemed surprising when it was first proposed—did this introduce an element of selfishness, or perhaps dilute or contradict the nurse's primary duty to the patient? In fact, it complements and reinforces that duty because nurses cannot provide adequate care to patients if they neglect their own needs—especially related to maintaining and protecting their own health and continuing their commitment to ongoing learning.

The 2001 Code of Ethics also introduced the idea that the nurse "participates in establishing, maintaining, and improving health care environments and conditions of employment conducive to the provision of quality health care." This emphasizes that nurses' ethical responsibilities apply not just to nurses providing direct patient care. It applies to nurses in all roles, including managerial roles, and calls for all nurses to take responsibility for ensuring positive nursing practice environments.

DIVERSITY IN HEALTH CARE

The United States has a racially, ethnically, and culturally diverse population. Health care outcomes vary dramatically according to the racial and ethnic backgrounds of people seeking care. Among the goals included in *Healthy People 2010,* a statement of the nation's health promotion and disease prevention goals, is the elimination of health disparities (Department of Health and Human Services, 2005).

Because of the diversity of the patient population and the lack of diversity in the health care labor force, over the past 20 years increased emphasis has been placed on the need for all health professionals to be culturally competent. Cultural competence has been defined within the Health Resources and Services Administration (HRSA) of the U.S. Department of Health and Human Services as a set of harmonious behaviors, attitudes, and policies that together enable a professional or an organization to work effectively in cross-cultural situations. HRSA actively seeks to increase the presence of health professionals of under-represented minority groups so as to better serve the needs of all patients (Department of Health and Human Services, 2006). In addition, the National Institutes of Health (NIH) established the National Center on Minority Health and Health Disparities in 1993, which introduced a national commitment and dialogue on health care needs, research, education, and funding, to address these disparities.

FACTORS INFLUENCING THE REGISTERED NURSE'S ROLE IN THE U.S. HEALTH CARE SYSTEM

The U.S. health care system is undergoing enormous change. Much of this change reflects concern with the rapid rise over the last 30 years in the cost of health care. This concern is increasingly expressed within government, the health professions, hospitals, the insurance industry, and by employers who provide health insurance to workers and families. The United States spends more money per capita on health care than any other developed nation. Yet, there is concern that many people are excluded from access to health care and that much of the money is not used as it was intended.

Nursing Shortage

The United States is experiencing a nursing shortage in most areas of the country. The shortage can be seen especially in critical care units, adult health units, the operating room, and the emergency department. Following a 5-year increase in applications to nursing schools, fewer individuals are entering nursing as a profession. This decline in nurses entering the profession combined with the anticipated retirement of a large number of nurses within the next 5 to 10 years is likely to contribute to the nursing shortage for the foreseeable future.

Shortened Stays

Among the ways that hospitals reduce the cost of the care they provide is the shortened stay. Patients may spend little time in the hospital, even if they are quite ill. Most surgery in the United States is now performed on an outpatient or same-day basis. New mothers are discharged within 24 hours of a vaginal delivery. People undergo much diagnostic testing as outpatients. They recuperate in their homes or in long-term care facilities. Terminally ill people often die at home with hospice support for their families.

In general, this means patients who are hospitalized are more ill, have more complex needs, and require more nursing care than was true a few years ago. Treatments and procedures that occurred in intensive care units in the past are now managed in regular medical or surgical units or in long-term care facilities. In addition, patients and their families need careful teaching to safely manage care after patients leave the hospital.

Efficiency in Staffing

In hospital settings, chief nursing officers are reorganizing their nursing staffs to be as cost-effective as possible. Nurses are often grouped into patient care teams with other types of health care workers, such as unlicensed assistive personnel, including nurse aides, certified nursing assistants, and patient care technicians. Because hospitalized patients have more nursing needs than was true in the past, and because of the nursing shortage, nurses find that their work load has increased over the last several years.

Expanded Home-Health and Community Services

Although most nurses work in hospital settings, more and more nurses are working in homecare and community settings. In those settings, it is routine for nurses to administer, or teach family members to administer, treatments and medications that were used only in critical care units a decade ago. For example, patients may go home with a central venous infusion or on a ventilator and require nurse visits once or more per day. Most hospitals now have homecare departments to organize nursing care for patients after they are discharged. Staff nurses also work closely with the homecare nurses to plan patient discharge.

Because hospitalized patients are so ill, and because nurses in homecare and community settings manage such complex health needs, nurses' ability to assess patients' health status and monitor change has never been so important. In addition, nurses increasingly coordinate patients' care by numerous departments or providers and fulfill the role of case manager. Because many different organizations or government agencies provide health insurance for most Americans, nurses must increasingly consider patients' individual insurance coverage in coordinating their care.

Advanced Technology

Another important stimulus for change in the U.S. health care delivery system is the common use of advanced technology for diagnosis, treatment, rehabilitation, and maintenance of patients who just a few years ago might not have survived. One example of this is the routine use by diabetic patients of electronic serum glucose-level testing devices. Other examples include the growing network of renal dialysis centers across the country, the increased use of home dialysis, and the expanding numbers of individuals who have undergone kidney transplants.

With increased technology has come more specialization in the provision of health care. Health care systems have become more complex associations of many departments or agencies. Patients sometimes feel that their care is fragmented and impersonal, and they look to nurses to help them understand their care and for care that meets their need for interpersonal communication.

Human Rights

Since the civil rights movement of the 1960s and 1970s, American society has become more keenly attuned to the autonomy and individual rights of all members of society, regardless of race, ethnicity, religious beliefs, gender, sexual orientation, or physical ability. Civil rights laws have shaped the way institutions deal with their employees and their patients.

The Patient Bill of Rights, adopted by the American Hospital Association and organizations that regulate health care, must be made available to patients in hospitals and nursing homes. This assures patients the right to be fully informed of all treatments, to refuse treatments, and to know the identity of all personnel involved in their care. The Patient Self Determination Act requires that the provider ask the patient about end-of-life decisions and documentation of a living will and power of attorney.

HIPAA Requirements

To improve the efficiency and effectiveness of the health care system, the Health Insurance Portability and Accountability Act of 1996 (HIPAA), Public Law 104–191, included provisions that required the Department of Health and Human Services (HHS) to adopt national standards that address the privacy of health information. The Privacy Rule implementing the law gives patients rights over their health information and sets rules and limits on who can look at and receive their health information. Protected health information includes:

- Information that doctors, nurses, and other health care providers put in the patient's medical record;
- Conversations that the primary care provider, nurses, and others have about the patient's care or treatment;
- Information about the patient that is in the health insurer's computer system;
- Billing information related to the patient; and
- Most other health information about the patient held by those who must follow this law, for example, health care providers and insurance plans.

Patients are asked to sign a form prior to admission or their receipt of health care indicating that the regulations governing HIPAA have been explained. Patients have the right to:

- Ask to see and get a copy of their health records;
- Have corrections added to their health information;
- Receive a notice that tells them how their health information may be used and shared;

- Decide if they want to give permission before their health information can be used or shared for certain purposes, such as for marketing;
- Get a report on when and why their health information was shared for certain purposes; and
- File a complaint with their provider or health insurance company or the U.S. government if they believe their rights are being denied or their health information is not being protected.

Patient health information cannot be used or shared without the patient's written permission except in cases where this law allows it. For example, without the patient's authorization, health care workers generally cannot give information to the patient's employer; use or share the patient's information for marketing or advertising purposes; or share private notes about the patient's health care.

Malpractice

The U.S. health care system has increasingly embraced a philosophy of self-care, or collaboration in care with patients and their families. Patients increasingly question their care if they believe their care is inadequate or inappropriate. They also have become more likely to use the legal system to address their grievances. In part, this may reflect the diminution in direct contact between patients and health care personnel and the increased use of technology.

Health care providers have turned to the strategies of quality control and risk management in addressing concerns related to the complexity and fragmentation of care and of legal risk, and nurses play a central role in quality assurance and risk management. Quality control refers to the examination of the care provided to a patient to ensure that it is of value and has not harmed the patient. Quality control includes such measures as the performance of health care providers, patient satisfaction, and patient outcomes, to name a few.

Risk management for health care institutions involves protection of the organization and individual providers from liability. The goals of a risk management program are to improve patient safety, to increase patient satisfaction, and to avoid risk. Risk control techniques are used to reduce patient errors.

NURSING ACROSS THE LIFE SPAN

Nurses in the United States provide care across the patient's life span—from prenatal care to palliative care at the end of life. There are four major areas of nursing practice: maternal/infant nursing; nursing of children (pediatric nursing); adult health nursing (medical–surgical nursing); and psychiatric/mental health nursing. Nursing practice in these four areas takes place in many different types of facilities—from critical care units to long-term care facilities and from in-patient settings to out-patient or clinic settings. No matter what the setting, nursing care can be divided into one of the four major areas.

Maternal/Infant Nursing

Maternal/infant nursing focuses on the care of childbearing women and their families through all stages of pregnancy and childbirth, as well as the first 4 weeks following birth. Maternal/infant nurses provide education about pregnancy; about the process of labor, birth, and recovery; and about parenting skills. They also promote health during childbearing, which can have a significant impact, not only on the health of individual women and their infants, but also on society.

Practice Settings

Throughout the prenatal period, nurses provide care for women in clinics and physician offices and teach classes to help families prepare for childbirth. Maternal/infant nurses also care for the family during labor and birth in hospitals, birthing centers, and in the home. Nurses with special education may provide intensive care for high-risk neonates in special care units (such as neonatal intensive care) and for high-risk mothers in antepartal units, in critical care obstetric units, or in the home.

Nurse Midwives

Maternity care has changed dramatically in the United States. Women now can choose a physician or a nurse midwife as their primary care provider. They can choose to have their birth in a hospital, in a birthing center, or in the home. Certified nurse midwives provide safe quality care. Women who choose nurse midwives as their primary care providers participate actively in childbirth decisions and receive fewer interventions, such as epidural analgesia for labor.

Family Centered Care

Maternity care in the United States is now family centered with fathers, significant others, grandparents, siblings, and friends present for labor and birth. Newborns remain with the mother and may breastfeed immediately after birth. Parents participate in the care of their infants in nurseries and in neonatal intensive care units.

Maternal nursing care is changing to single-room maternity care, in which a woman labors, gives birth, and recovers in the same room—the entire stay for birth may occur in the same room. In some hospitals, central nurseries have been eliminated and babies stay in the room with their mothers. Instead of having one nurse care for the baby and another nurse care for the mother, some hospitals have one nurse care for both as a unit. Many hospitals employ lactation consultants to assist mothers with breastfeeding. Discharge of a mother and baby within 24 to 48 hours after the birth is common practice and results in the growing need for follow-up or home care to ensure that the mother, infant, and family are adjusting at home.

Nursing of Children

Nursing of children, or pediatric nursing, in the United States focuses on preventing illness and injury in children. Nurses working in this specialty area assist children to obtain optimal levels of health and assist with the rehabilitation of ill children. Pediatric nurses provide direct nursing care to children and families and play an important role in minimizing the stress experienced by children and their families when children are ill.

Family Centered Care

Most pediatric nurses and pediatric health care facilities adhere to the philosophy of family centered nursing. This philosophy of care recognizes the central role of the family in the child's life and includes the family in the child's plan of care and its delivery. Research shows that when families are incorporated into the child's plan of care the physical and psychosocial health of the child improves. As a result, family centered nursing evolved to maintain the relationships between hospitalized children and their families.

In family centered care, all family members are involved with a child recovering from illness or injury. The pediatric nurse who practices family centered care provides for the emotional, social, and developmental needs of both the child and the family.

Role of the Pediatric Nurse

A goal of pediatric nursing is to restore the ill child to the appropriate developmental level of functioning and to prevent injury and illness in the child. This focus requires the pediatric nurse to have a broad knowledge base that includes understanding the culture at large, being aware of health and illness issues related to children, and maintaining a wide range of clinical competencies. Pediatric nurses work with children in general hospitals, children's hospitals, the home, schools, physician offices, psychiatric centers, summer camps, and in other community settings.

Range of Pediatric Nursing

Pediatric nurses need to be aware of the various stages of development to provide age-appropriate care to both sick and well children. Pediatric nursing encompasses the care of children from infancy (birth to 1 year) through adolescence (12 to 19 years) or later. Infancy is characterized by a rapid period of growth and change. It is at this time that attachments to family members and other caregivers are formed and trust develops.

The toddler stage of development (1 to 3 years of age) is the time in which children develop motor ability, coordination, and sensory skills. Toddlers begin to develop a sense of self and a growing independence. The preschool years (3 to 6 years) are a time of continued physiological, psychological, and cognitive growth. Children in this age group begin to care for themselves, become interested in playing with other children, and begin to develop a concept of who they are.

The school-age child (6 to 12 years) is generally interested in achievement, focuses on the ability to read and write, and enjoys completing academic coursework. It is during this stage that the child's understanding of the world broadens. During adolescence (12 to 19 years) physiological maturation occurs and preparation for becoming an adult takes place. Adolescence is the transition between childhood and adulthood.

Adult Health Nursing

The focus of adult health or medical/surgical nursing is on the adult patient with acute or chronic illness in any health care setting. In the United States, nurses who work in adult health nursing must have a broad knowledge base that includes not only nursing but also the biological, psychological, and social sciences. Adult health nurses must have an understanding of the social, cultural, psychological, physical, spiritual, and economic factors that affect the patient's health and health care. Such knowledge is required because the patients for whom adult health nurses care range in age from 18 years to more than 100 years, and their health problems are often complex.

The overall outcome of care for adult health nursing is the achievement of an optimal level of wellness and prevention of illness. Adult health nurses practice in various roles and functions within a number of health care settings. They serve as patient caregivers and patient advocates. They are usually involved in care planning and education and serve as managers and coordinators of care.

Employment Settings

Adult health nurses function in many settings in health care institutions, including critical care units and medical surgical units. They work in positions in long-term care and in the community. Adult health nurses also are involved in home care, providing follow-up to patients who have been discharged from the hospital setting. Increasingly, adult health nurses are working in ambulatory health care settings, such as physician offices, hospitals or free-standing out-patient clinics, independent surgical centers, and health maintenance organizations. The focus of ambulatory care is on health promotion, illness prevention, short-term treatment, and follow-up for existing health problems.

Gerontological Nursing

When the patient is older than 65 years, adult health nurses also need a strong background in gerontology or care of the elderly. Nurses today will care for more adults over 65 than any other patient population. They will provide this care in hospitals, community health centers, senior centers, long-term care facilities, and patients' homes.

Gerontological nurses care for the physical and psychosocial needs of older adults. They focus on maximizing the patient's functional abilities, as well as promoting, maintaining, and restoring his or her physical and mental health. Science has shown that the human body changes with aging. Therefore, nurses engaged in gerontological nursing need to modify how they assess, plan, deliver, and evaluate nursing care in order to provide the safest, highest quality care possible to the older adult patient (and that addresses the changing needs of the patient).

The gerontological nurse must consider the physiologic changes associated with aging, the way in which illness presents itself, the manner in which the human body responds to treatment, and which treatments are appropriate. The nurse's care planning and care delivery must address such issues as the functional decline in hospitalized older adults, the older adult's nutritional needs and interventions, and appropriate medication administration and teaching.

Psychiatric/Mental Health Nursing

Psychiatric nursing emerged in the early 1950s in the United States. Psychiatric nursing is an interpersonal process that promotes and maintains patient (also known as client) behavior that contributes to the integrated functioning of mind and body. The psychiatric/mental health nurse establishes therapeutic relationships with clients and uses his or her own personality and communication skills to form and maintain these relationships.

The client may be an individual, family, group, organization, or community. Traditional settings in which psychiatric nurses practice include psychiatric hospitals, community mental health centers, psychiatric units in general hospitals, residential facilities, and private practice. In the United States, there has been a move to shift the care of mentally ill patients from institutions to community settings. The psychiatric nurse bases nursing practice on the psychosocial and biophysical sciences as well as on the theories of personality and human behavior.

The role of the psychiatric nurse encompasses clinical competence, client–family advocacy, interdisciplinary collaboration, social accountability, and legal–ethical practice. The primary objectives of psychiatric nursing are:

- To facilitate the maximum development of the mental health of the individual who has psychiatric/mental health issues and problems;
- To promote the mental health of clients;
- To rehabilitate patients and clients so that as many as possible can live full lives in community settings; and
- To support those with psychiatric/mental health disorders already living in the community.

Psychiatric nurses achieve these goals by incorporating the concepts of primary, secondary, and tertiary prevention.

Primary Prevention

Primary prevention in psychiatric nursing comprises the prevention of illness in a community by changing the causes of the illness before harm is done. For psychiatric nurses this involves teaching about principles of mental health; effecting changes in living conditions, poverty levels, and education; working with families; and making appropriate referrals before mental illness occurs.

Secondary Prevention

Secondary prevention involves reducing mental illness by early detection and treatment of the problem. For psychiatric nurses, secondary prevention includes intake screening, home visits, suicide prevention services, crisis intervention, and other counseling interventions.

Tertiary Prevention

Tertiary prevention entails reducing the impairment from an illness. For psychiatric nurses this includes promoting vocational training and rehabilitation, organizing programs to ease the transition from hospital to community, and providing partial hospitalization for patients.

NURSING PROCESS

Nurses in the United States are taught a step-by-step, problem-solving approach to determining and meeting their patients' needs. This problem-solving approach is called the nursing process. Not only is it used within the practice setting, but it also is integrated throughout both the CGFNS and the U.S. licensure examinations. There are five basic steps to this problem-solving approach: assessment, analysis or diagnosis, planning, implementation, and evaluation.

Assessment

Assessment refers to establishing an information base. It includes gathering subjective and objective information, confirming data, and communicating findings. In the assessment phase, the nurse gathers information about the patient that is needed to plan appropriate nursing care.

Ideally, an initial nursing assessment is conducted on admission of the patient and is comprehensive in nature. In reality, the urgency of the patient's needs at the time of the initial assessment (e.g., a patient admitted to the emergency department) determines how much time can be taken to complete the assessment. Generally, the comprehensive assessment is done at the time of admission, and an abbreviated assessment is done on a daily basis. The nurse's assessment of the patient's status is critical because all other steps in the nursing process are based on this information.

Source of Information

In preparing to assess a specific patient, the nurse may have access to information from other health care professionals, such as the primary care provider (physician or nurse practitioner), the social worker, or other nurses. The nurse may have access to the patient's record containing information about past health care or the assessment and treatment provided by other health professionals.

The nurse also may have an opportunity to talk with the patient, or, if the patient is unable, family members about why this patient has come for health care. There may be witnesses to a sudden illness or injury who can provide background information. It is important for the nurse to use as much information as can be found from these sources so that time with the patient can be used most efficiently. Two broad types of information are gathered in a nursing assessment: objective information and subjective information.

Objective Information

Objective information is the information gathered through use of the senses, that is, sight, hearing, touch, and smell. Laboratory and diagnostic test results and assessments by other members of the health care team are included as objective information, even though the nurse usually does not gather this information directly. Objective data also is obtained through the use of diagnostic equipment, such as thermometers, stethoscopes, cardiac monitors, and central venous lines. What makes this information objective is that it can be confirmed by other people using the same equipment or the same procedures.

Subjective Information

Subjective information refers to what the patient, family members, or witnesses say about the patient's condition. It is what they think, feel, remember, or believe. The nurse cannot observe this type of information directly. This is how the nurse learns about the patient's history, the development of a specific problem, what the patient tried to do about the problem before seeking health care, and the patient's and family's understanding, beliefs, and feelings, about the health problem. This information is part of the nursing history.

Nursing History

The nursing history also includes general background information about the patient's past health and the health of family members. The nurse will ask the patient questions reviewing the body systems, such as the respiratory or circulatory systems. The nurse also will assess the patient's usual activities of daily living and how they may have been altered by the current illness.

The nurse also will review the patient's growth and development, history of coping with crises in the past, and sources of support. The way the nurse, staff, or significant others react to the patient may be important in addressing the patient's health needs. The nurse's concerns are whether or not the patient, the family, and the health care team are able to meet the patient's health needs in the patient's environment and how the illness or injury alters the patient's ability to function.

Physical Assessment

Nurses in the United States are taught physical assessment skills, and it is expected that they will assess each patient thoroughly upon or near the time of admission and then as often as needed, depending upon change in the patient's condition. These repeated assessments are usually much briefer than the initial assessment.

Initially, the nurse will thoroughly assess the patient's status in relation to the problem that made him or her seek health care. In addition, if the patient's urgency of need does not preclude it, the nurse will assess each body system. As the nurse performs the assessment, the nurse will note how the patient's status conforms to norm for his or her developmental stage.

Communicating Findings

The objective and subjective assessments and nursing history must be communicated to other members of the health care team to be most useful to the patient. This is usually done by means of the patient's chart and through the report that is given to on-coming staff (shift report).

Most institutions have developed standardized forms used to record the nursing assessment. The information must be recorded clearly and accurately. Direct quotes by the patient should be marked as such and used whenever possible. The information should be both complete and brief. This is not the stage in the nursing process for the nurse to convey what he or she thinks about the patient's situation—it is the stage of data collection.

Analysis

Analysis, also known as diagnosis, refers to the nurse's identification of actual or potential health care needs or problems based on the nursing assessment. Analysis includes interpretation of the data collected, formulation of nursing diagnoses, and communication of the nurse's analysis.

Once the nurse has completed the initial subjective and objective patient assessment, the nurse will begin to develop the plan of nursing care. At this point, the nurse must reflect upon all of the information gathered about the patient. The analysis step of the nursing process is the point at which the nurse organizes information and makes initial conclusions about the patient's status. These conclusions are the nursing diagnoses.

Nursing Diagnoses

To identify the nursing diagnoses, the nurse will note particularly those aspects of patient status that deviate from what is normal for a person of the patient's developmental status or that reflect developmental change. Based on these data and what the patient has said about his or her response to the current illness, injury, or developmental transitions, the nurse will consider how well the patient's needs are being met and how the patient's ability to function has been altered.

Unlike the medical diagnosis of a disease and the pathological changes it causes, nursing diagnoses focus on the patient's ability to cope with, and adapt to, his or her developmental status, illness, or injury. The nursing diagnosis will include the category label for the patient's response, and it will state whether the response is actual or potential. It will briefly state the observation that led the nurse to a particular conclusion, and it will identify the physical or psychosocial process to which the response is related.

The patient's nursing diagnoses reflect his or her current health status. They may vary frequently during the course of an illness. This is different from the medical diagnosis, which remains the same until the individual recovers or dies. To be useful to the patient, the nursing assessment must be documented, and nursing diagnoses must be reported to the health care team.

Nursing Diagnosis Classification

Many institutions have adopted the North American Nursing Diagnosis Association (NANDA) classification of human responses to illnesses and developmental or situational crises. An example of a nursing diagnosis using the NANDA terminology is: Alteration in comfort (pain) related to fourth-degree perineal tear during delivery as evidenced by patient's verbalization of pain, identification of pain as a 9 on a scale of 1–10, and patient's tearful expression.

Planning

The planning phase of the nursing process refers to prioritizing the nursing diagnoses, setting goals for meeting patient needs, and designing strategies for achieving patient goals. During the planning phase the nurse addresses these three questions:

1. What is to be done about the nursing diagnoses?
2. How is it to be done?
3. When is it to be done?

The answers to these questions establish the nursing care plan.

Nursing Care Plan

The nursing care plan is a written document initiated by one nurse so that other nursing staff on the unit know what nursing care the patient requires and when and how it is to be provided. Each nurse who cares for the patient may modify the care plan as the patient's status changes or as ways to make care more effective are discovered.

In addition to care indicated by the nursing diagnoses, nursing care related to the physician's diagnosis and treatment also is included on the care plan. There are several activities that the nurse must perform in the planning step of the nursing process. These planning activities are usually done simultaneously and include:

- Setting priorities,
- Establishing long-term and short-term goals and objectives,
- Determining outcome criteria,
- Developing the plan of care and modifying it as needed,
- Collaborating with health care team members in planning care, and
- Communicating the nursing care plan.

Setting Priorities

Setting priorities means deciding the relative urgency of attending to each nursing diagnosis. In deciding the order in which the nursing diagnoses should be addressed, the nurse will consider the patient's physiological needs, patient and family preferences and feelings of urgency about a given problem, the overall treatment plan for the patient, the demands of the total case load, and hospital or health care agency policies.

Establishing Long- and Short-Term Goals and Objectives

Establishing long- and short-term goals and objectives is crucial to the analysis phase of the nursing process. *Goals* refer to outcomes of care. *Objectives* are the steps that must be accomplished for the goal to be achieved. The objectives may change frequently as the patient progresses toward achievement of the goals of care.

Care Mapping. Many acute care facilities, such as hospitals, now plan care using a critical pathway model. This means for a specific illness or injury, the patient is expected to have a certain length of admission. During each day, the patient is expected to meet specific objectives to accomplish established short-term goals reflecting the patient's medical status, day of admission, and preparation for discharge.

The patient's goals, objectives, and status are reviewed daily to ensure that the patient is progressing as expected or to determine if the patient has additional health needs or problems. This approach to planning care increases the efficiency of hospitals and reduces wasted in-patient days.

Patient Goals. Long-term goals refer to outcomes that are expected upon follow-up or a regular check-up, or at a later developmental stage. Short-term goals refer to outcomes expected when an acute illness is resolved. For example, "The patient will attain height and weight at or above the 50th percentile by age by the second birthday" is an appropriate long-term goal for a low birth-weight baby. A short-term goal might be, "The patient will attain a weight of 2.5 kilograms by the fourth week of dietary modification."

Goals of care should be patient-focused. They are outcomes the nurse is assisting the patient to achieve. The goals, particularly the long-term goals, will guide discharge planning. Patient teaching to prepare for discharge will address the goals.

Objectives. Objectives, which are steps the patient will take in achieving the goal, are also written from the patient's perspective. For example, "The patient will give a return demonstration of a baby bath before discharge from the postpartum unit." The goals and objectives must be realistic, acceptable to the patient and family, and in agreement with the overall treatment plan for the patient.

Determining Outcome Criteria

As the goals and objectives of care are established, concrete ways to evaluate whether or not they are met are identified for each. This includes the establishment of deadlines by which goals and objectives are to be met. Criteria and deadlines reflect both the patient's health needs or problems and length-of-stay guidelines for a particular patient's condition.

There are several reasons for anticipating to what degree and by when the patient will achieve goals and objectives. One reason is to ensure that the patient will progress toward discharge in a timely manner. Another is to motivate the patient and the nurse to keep progressing toward their achievement. However, criteria and deadlines must be realistic. Failure to meet an objective at the expected time can be discouraging, and if the patient does not achieve objectives or goals, they must be reviewed. It may be that the patient's health needs or problems were more complex than the nurse realized; that the deadlines, goals, or objectives were not reasonable; or that referral to additional supportive services is required. The nurse will be guided by experience and by the patient assessments in determining outcome criteria and deadlines.

Developing the Plan of Care and Modifying It as Needed

Once the goals and objectives have been established with outcome criteria, the nurse identifies appropriate nursing care activities (interventions) and selects those that will be most effective in helping the patient meet the objectives in the anticipated time. The plan of care will be more effective if the patient and family as well as other health care team members are involved in its development.

The plan of care needs to reflect consideration of the patient's developmental status, gender, culture, and religious values. Moreover, each patient is unique, and what works best for one person may not be the preferred strategy with another. The plan of care incorporates concern for the patient's safety, comfort, and optimal functioning.

The nursing care plan will reflect various types of nursing care activities: monitoring patient status, nursing treatments, instruction of patient and family, and the referral of patient or family to other sources of assistance. The nurse may have to identify alternate interventions if the ones initially selected do not result in the meeting of the objectives of the care of the patient within the allotted time.

Nursing Orders. The nursing care plan includes nursing orders. Nursing orders describe the nursing care activities to be undertaken for or with the patient in order to meet each objective, including how the activities should be carried out, at what time, and for how long. Nursing orders must be compatible with orders written by the physician and others because they must fit into the overall treatment plan. Examples of nursing orders include:

- Offer 300 ml. of fluid at least every two hours while patient is awake for a total of 2400 ml. intake every 24 hours.
- Have patient perform return demonstration of fundal massage during postpartum admission assessment.
- Perform range-of-motion exercises while bathing patient.

Collaborating With Health Care Team Members in Planning Care

Development of the plan of care for the patient includes identification of health or social service resources available to the patient and family. These resources should enter into the development of the overall plan of care for the patient and may comprise additions to the care plan as needed.

In addition, the nurse plans nursing team assignments to most suitably match team members with patients according to their needs identified in the care plan. Finally, the nurse coordinates care provided to patients by members of the health care team.

Communicating the Nursing Care Plan

The nursing care plan helps the patient only if it is communicated. Careful documentation of the plan of care requires that nursing goals and objectives be identified for each nursing diagnosis with the deadlines by which they are to be achieved. For each objective, nursing orders are listed with the times they are to be carried out. Nursing activities that must be performed based upon medical orders also are listed and scheduled.

In addition, the plan of care is reported to the health care team and discussed with the patient and his/her family. Because the plan is developed in collaboration with the patient, family, and other health team members, the plan should be reviewed periodically with everyone.

Implementation

During this step in the nursing process, the nurse actually initiates and completes the actions necessary to accomplish the short-term and long-term goals. The nurse also provides the nursing care that was planned to the patient. This includes organizing and managing the patient's care, counseling and teaching the patient and family, providing care to achieve established goals, supervising and coordinating the care provided by other nursing and health care personnel, and communicating nursing interventions.

Delegation of Care

The nurse may give nursing care personally or may delegate aspects of the nursing care to other nursing staff members. If the nurse assigns tasks to others, the nurse is still responsible for making sure that the nursing care is given according to the nursing orders on the care plan. Patient care conferences may be arranged to obtain updates on the care plan and to provide more consistent, focused care delivery.

Family Centered Care

Nursing care is focused on assisting patients and families to maintain optimal functioning and includes encouraging patients and families to adhere to the treatment regimen. The nurse may facilitate patient relationships with family members as well as health care team members.

Patients and their families need to be informed as to the patient's health status, and they require teaching of correct principles, procedures, and techniques for health maintenance and health promotion. Care is modified in accord with patients' preferences, needs, or problems. Also, patients and their families are referred to appropriate resources when necessary.

Nurses strive to provide an environment conducive to the patient's attainment of the goals of care. Patients and families need anticipatory guidance prior to surgery, childbirth, or other procedures, particularly those that are invasive. Anticipatory guidance helps the patient and family to understand what will be happening during these interventions and what to expect before, during, and after the procedures.

Communication of Findings

Nursing interventions must be communicated to ensure safe, coordinated care for the patient. Nursing interventions and the patient's responses to them are recorded, and staff are provided complete, accurate reports on the status of their assigned patients.

Evaluation

Evaluation is the last step in the nursing process. It is an ongoing activity throughout the period in which nursing care is given and follow-up care provided. The nurse will continually ask whether or not the goals of nursing care have been met. Over time, the nurse will assess the reasonableness of the short-term and long-term goals, the objectives, and the patient's progress in meeting them.

Patient Response to Care

The nurse will examine patient responses to care, including both those that are expected and those that are unexpected. The nurse also will assess the overall effect of therapeutic interventions on the patient and family, including whether the patient is experiencing any new problems as a result of the nursing care.

The nurse will evaluate whether or not the patient and family understand the information they receive. In addition, the nurse continually assesses the patient's and family's ability to monitor the patient's status and carry out procedures. The patient's and family's self-care ability is an important factor in health maintenance and health promotion, recuperation, or death with dignity.

The nurse will also evaluate whether the nursing care is keeping the patient as safe and as comfortable as possible. The nurse will need to evaluate the patient's use of time, energy, supplies, and equipment in carrying out the nursing care. The discovery of new information about the patient may require that the nurse revise the plan of care. Each nurse who provides nursing care to the patient following the nursing care plan will consider these patient outcomes and make or suggest appropriate modifications in the nursing care plan.

Evaluation may be the most important part of the nursing process because it answers the question, "Is the nursing care helping the patient achieve the objectives and goals of care?" This allows nurses to use their time as efficiently as possible because care that does not facilitate a patient's progress is not continued.

Communication of Results

Evaluation must be communicated for it to be useful to the patient. Patient responses to therapy, care, and teaching are documented and reported to relevant members of the health care team. In addition, caregivers' and staff members' responses are communicated when they suggest modification of the plan of care.

Summary of the Nursing Process

The steps in the nursing process are described as though they follow one after the other in sequence. In reality, nurses do not think this way. In many instances, several steps are carried out at the same time. Both assessment and evaluation are ongoing. Whenever the nurse provides nursing care, he or she will ask whether it is effective. If it is not, then the objectives, plan, and nursing activities need to be changed. All of the steps in the nursing process overlap and cannot be considered as separate and distinct.

The ideal situation is one in which the patient can participate throughout the nursing process. If the patient is too ill, too upset, comatose, or confused, this will not be possible. It may be possible to include family members in the process of planning, giving, and evaluating care, but there will be times when the nurse must decide what the goals, objectives, and plan of care should be.

SUMMARY

Adjusting to nursing practice in the United States includes becoming familiar with the ways in which the profession sets its own standards, identifies the scope of nursing practice, and determines how care is to be provided. It also requires familiarity with the laws and regulations regulating nursing practice in the state in which you are licensed. Like all other aspects of adjusting to living and practicing in the United States, this is a process of acquiring, using, and assimilating new knowledge.

REFERENCES

American Board of Nursing Specialties. (2000). *Accreditation of nursing specialties accreditation program.* Retrieved February 16, 2009, from http://www.nursingcertifica tion.org/exam_programs.htm

American Nurses Association. (2001). *Code of ethics for nurses with interpretive statements.* Silver Spring, MD: Author.

American Nurses Association. (2003). *Nursing's social policy statement* (2nd ed.). Silver Spring, MD: Author.

American Nurses Association. (2004). *Nursing: Scope and standards of practice.* Silver Spring, MD: Author.

American Nurses Association & National Council of State Boards of Nursing. (2006). *Joint statement on delegation.* Retrieved January 28, 2009, from https://www.ncsbn. org/Joint_statement.pdf

American Nurses Credentialing Center. (2009). *Certification: Frequently asked questions.* Retrieved February 16, 2009, from http://www.nursecredentialing.org/cert/FAQ.html

Department of Health and Human Services. (2005). *Healthy people 2010.* Retrieved April 26, 2009, from http://www.healthypeople.gov/Publications/Cornerstone.pdf

Department of Health and Human Services. (2006). *What is cultural competence?* Office of Minority Health. Retrieved April 26, 2009, from http://www.omhrc.gov/templates/browse.aspx?lvl=2&lvlID=11

National Commission on Certifying Agencies. (2009). *NCCA accreditation.* Retrieved February 16, 2009, from http://www.noca.org/Resources/NCCAAccreditation/tabid/82/Default.aspx

National Council of State Boards of Nursing. (2008). *Consensus model for APRN regulation: Licensure, accreditation, certification & education.* Retrieved February 16, 2009, from https://www.ncsbn.org/7_23_08_Consensue_APRN_Final.pdf

New York State Education Department. (2002). *Abandonment in nursing.* Retrieved January 28, 2009, from http://www.op.nysed.gov/nurseabandonment.htm

Styles, M. M., Schumann, M. J., Bickford, C., & White, K. M. (2008). *Specialization and credentialing in nursing revisited.* Silver Spring, MD: Author.

8

Communicating in the U.S. Health Care System

CATHERINE R. DAVIS
DONNA R. RICHARDSON

In This Chapter

Legal Basis for U.S. Language Proficiency Requirements

Interpersonal Skills

Assertiveness

Nonverbal Communication

Idioms, Slang, and Abbreviations

Which Language to Use

Summary

Keywords

Acculturation program: A system of procedures or activities that has the specific purpose of training individuals to understand another culture and its practices.

Assertiveness: Ability to state one's position positively and in a self-confident manner.

Cross-cultural communication: Interaction between two or more individuals of different cultures.

Cultural conflicts: Disagreements that arise due to misunderstandings in communication and personal interpretations of words and actions.

Focus group: A small group of people who are questioned about their opinions as part of research.

Idiom: An expression of speech whose meaning is translated figuratively rather than literally.

Jargon: An informal language used by people who work together within a specific occupation or profession or within a common interest group.

Role-playing: Practicing how you will respond in a situation by playing the part you will take or that of another person, for example, practicing your interaction with a physician who has written an order that you must question.

Slang: Highly informal words or expressions that are not considered standard in the language.

The ability to communicate effectively in the health care setting is a skill that is not only critical to safe practice but also highly valued. This chapter will focus on the interpersonal and language challenges that many foreign-educated nurses face as they enter practice in the United States.

Communication—the exchange of ideas or information through spoken words, writing, or gestures—is important to safe nursing practice. In the United States, English is the language used in health care settings and in nursing practice. The perception of foreign-educated nurses as competent providers of care in the United States has been linked, in part, to their ability to communicate in English and to understand verbal and written English communication in order to ensure safe patient care.

LEGAL BASIS FOR U.S. LANGUAGE PROFICIENCY REQUIREMENTS

The United States relies on foreign-educated nurses to supplement its workforce in times of shortage. However, previous nursing shortages and their corresponding recruitment patterns have not prepared the health care community for the magnitude of diverse backgrounds from which nurses migrate today. Most nurses who came to the United States during previous nursing shortages were from the Philippines, the United Kingdom, or Canada. However, due to evolving migration patterns and the expansion of nursing education globally, nurses now come to the United States from all over the world.

With nurses entering the U.S. health workforce with such diverse backgrounds, the U.S. government, through the 1996 Illegal Immigration Reform and Immigrant Responsibility Act, mandated that health care professionals seeking to practice in the United States demonstrate a certain level of proficiency in written and spoken English. The regulations implementing the 1996 Act identified the accepted English language tests and score requirements for certain health care professions, including nursing. The required English language proficiency examinations and their score requirements may be found in chapter 3, Table 3.1, or on the CGFNS Web site: http://www.cgfns.org/files/pdf/req/vs-requirements.pdf.

One of the requirements of the CGFNS VisaScreen program, which is required for nurses seeking occupational visas to practice in the United States, is the successful demonstration of English language proficiency as required by the 1996 law. Currently, a registered or practical nurse coming to work in the United States must achieve the government-mandated scores on one of the sets of English language proficiency examinations to obtain the VisaScreen certificate. This certificate must be presented at the embassy or consular office at the time of your visa interview.

In addition to the federal government's English language mandate, State Boards of Nursing are requiring more documentation of English language proficiency to ensure that the health care team, patients, and families receive the health information they need to make important health decisions. Patient complaints and poor patient outcomes are reinforcing the need for improved skills in communication, which can be an especially challenging issue for nurses whose first language is other than English. In fact, some states believe that lack of language proficiency contributes to medication errors and failures in multi-disciplinary communication. For that reason, many states are requiring nurses to take and pass English language proficiency examinations or to submit a CGFNS Certification Program certificate or VisaScreen certificate (see chapter 4, "The Role of CGFNS International").

INTERPERSONAL SKILLS

Health communication has recently received increased visibility in the United States, with many health organizations conducting research and producing literature related to this topic. One objective of *Healthy People 2010*, a set of national health goals published by the U.S. Department of Health and Human Services (2008), is to "increase the proportion of persons who report that their health care providers have satisfactory communication skills." Effective communication of health care information is especially important because the U.S. health care system places increased responsibility on individuals for their own health and wellness.

Cross-Cultural Conflicts

Increasing globalization and global mobility are bringing new immigrants to the United States from a wide array of countries. As a result, nurses in the United States are interacting with people—both patients and colleagues—from many different cultures. Culture helps to shape an individual's values, beliefs, and identity. However, **cultural conflicts** can arise due to misunderstandings in communication and personal interpretations. In the workplace some of these differences can relate to the perception of time, to the way work is organized and completed, and to the way in which communications and interactions are managed.

Cross-cultural conflicts in nursing can be minimized or prevented by learning more about the individual cultures of coworkers and patients. Conflicts also may be minimized by a willingness and openness in sharing personal and professional experiences and practices. Many hospitals are providing opportunities for such interaction, which can help to reduce cultural conflict if U.S.-educated and foreign-educated nurses are willing to share their stories, discuss their similarities and differences, and develop a relationship built on respect.

Cross-Cultural Communication

It seems that in the workplace, at least, people are often more comfortable interacting with others who share the same cultural or ethnic background, especially where language is involved. This may provide a "comfort zone" or safe environment, especially for newly arrived immigrants. The way in which we communicate is probably influenced most by the culture in which we were reared, therefore, the foundation of *successful* **cross-cultural communication** is having some degree of understanding of each other's culture and its norms. This basic understanding can reduce the anxiety of living, working, and communicating in a culturally diverse country, such as the United States. One foreign-educated nurse very eloquently addressed the topic of cultural challenges and communication during a CGFNS (2000) **focus group:**

> No one ever told me about in North America, the diversity. Here in North America there is a very wide diversity of cultures. The gays, the single mothers, teen pregnancies, those with addiction—they are accepted here. But in many countries and cultures, like India, Asia, the Middle East, these are not accepted. I'm not saying they don't exist, but they're not brought to light. So the foreign-educated nurse has not seen these things, and here, nursing is based on community. A foreign-educated nurse needs to understand the diversity of culture. This is very important, because when [she] approaches the client or patient, the nurse needs to be unbiased and not judge.

Tips to Promote Cross-Cultural Communication

The facility in which you work, and even the unit to which you are assigned, also will have its own culture, its own norms, and its own values and rules. Cross-cultural interaction has its challenges, and it is important to remember that you may not always be successful in communicating. However, you can minimize the stress of cross-cultural communication by:

- *Taking the initiative to ask* if you are unsure of what is expected of you, or what a colleague, supervisor, physician or patient is trying to explain to you.
- *Making sure you understand* what was said by summarizing what you heard for clarification and accuracy. For example, you might say to a colleague or patient, "This is what I understood you to have said … Am I correct?" You should confirm the intended meaning of both verbal and nonverbal communication to prevent misunderstandings.
- *Finding an intermediary* who can interact with you and your patient or colleagues if messages are unclear. Your mentor/ preceptor, or some other person you trust, might serve in this role.
- *Requesting feedback* by asking a colleague or patient, "Can you understand clearly what I'm saying?" Feedback can help to correct misconceptions so that both parties have the same understanding.

In a study of foreign-educated nurses in the U.S. workforce, CGFNS (2002) found that many of the nurses had communication difficulties in the workplace but were taking steps to increase their language proficiency. The most common issues were talking on the telephone, talking with physicians, and talking with patients and their families. Talking on the telephone was particularly challenging when speaking with a physician for whom English also was a second language.

Role-Playing

One of the suggestions for remedying the language challenges of foreign-educated nurses was **role-playing.** Many of the nurses reported practicing communicating with a "physician," both in person and on the telephone, during their orientation to the facility. Many also role-played situations in which they had to communicate with "patients" and their "families." The more they practiced, the easier the communication became when the nurses experienced these simulated communications in the actual practice setting.

ASSERTIVENESS

Assertiveness is the ability to honestly express your opinions, feelings, concerns, and attitudes in a way that does not infringe on another's rights and does not cause you and others undue anxiety. Assertive communication allows both parties to maintain self-respect.

Physician Interactions

In the United States, nurses see themselves as being colleagues of physicians, rather than as being subservient to them, because it is an integral part of their education. Nurses interact frequently with physicians, discussing patient conditions, treatment options, and personal observations. Nurses are required to confirm physician orders and will question physician orders if they believe they are in error.

In fact, nurses in the United States are legally and ethically accountable for their own actions. Nurses must question the actions of doctors and other professionals if they pose a danger to patient care. This even includes refusing to carry out a physician's orders and notifying the appropriate supervisor if the nurse believes the orders are unsafe. Such actions require assertiveness, tact, and negotiation, all of which necessitate proficiency in the use of the English language.

Patient Interactions

Interacting with patients also may require assertiveness. In the United States, the nurse is not only a provider of care, but also a teacher, an intermediary between patient and physician, and a patient advocate. To fulfill these roles, the nurse must have not only good verbal communication skills but also good documentation skills to ensure continuity of care, patient understanding of care, and maintenance of legal records, such as the patient's chart.

As nurses work in more intense and complex situations, the need for assertiveness increases. Nurses who are not assertive in their communications often feel as if they have little or no control over a situation. Becoming more assertive can lead to more respect—and more positive responses to your nursing knowledge and experience—from patients and coworkers.

Nonassertive Communication

Assertiveness is a skill that requires practice. It can be difficult to give your opinion, to express your needs, and to confront the behavior of others if you have not been encouraged to do so. Being assertive will take you out of your comfort zone, especially when you first attempt it. That is why many nurses move from being passive in their interactions to being aggressive in making their needs known—and then finally become assertive, with practice.

What are some of the signs that you are *not* being assertive? You are considered nonassertive in the United States if you:

- Consider yourself to be less knowledgeable or less capable than others, despite your education;
- Avoid eye contact;
- Don't take a position on issues—even when a situation dictates that you should;
- Try to prevent conflict at all costs;
- Try not to be the decision maker;
- Are unable to say "no"; or
- Try not to be noticed in work or social situations.

Assertive Communication

Assertiveness requires that you express your thoughts, opinions, and feelings without offending others. You can develop your assertiveness by following these recommendations:

- Use "I" statements instead of "You" statements when interacting. For example, when you disagree with someone, instead of saying, "You are not correct," try saying, "I appreciate your opinion—and I have a different perspective." Then calmly state that perspective.
- Use assertive body language. Face the person with whom you are attempting to communicate, keep your voice calm, stand up straight, and be aware of your facial expressions.
- Be factual and not judgmental. Do not apologize for your opinion.
- Make clear and direct requests that do not encourage the other person to say "no." For example, if a patient on the psychiatric unit tries to avoid participating in group therapy, instead of saying, "Would you like to go to therapy today?" say, "I'll be taking you to therapy at 10 o'clock this morning."

Support Systems

Sometimes becoming assertive requires a support system. Practice with trusted friends and family. Start with small steps. If you find that you hesitate to speak up in meetings at work, find out what the meeting agenda is beforehand and decide to speak on a topic that is of interest to you. Try to choose a topic early in the agenda so that you don't have to think about your response during the entire meeting. Formulate your opinion, then practice speaking it out loud so that when you are in the meeting, you will feel less nervous and will be able to voice your opinion. Act confidently—even if you do not feel confident.

NONVERBAL COMMUNICATION

Communication is composed of two interrelated dimensions: verbal communication and nonverbal communication. The key components of verbal communication are sound, words, speaking, and language.

Nonverbal communication includes such attributes as facial expression, eye contact, touching, tone of voice, posture, and physical distance maintained during communication. Even silence can be a form of nonverbal communication, and it often can have a greater impact than the spoken word. Nonverbal communication tends to express inner feelings, is more genuine, and is less likely to be as controlled as the spoken word.

It is important for the nurse to be aware of the role of nonverbal communication in the work setting because others make judgments about competence and character by observing nonverbal behaviors. Body posture can be an indicator of your self-confidence, your energy, or your fatigue. Facial expressions can intentionally or unintentionally convey emotions, attitudes, and internal feelings. Your eyes can indicate positive or negative relationships.

Eye Contact

People tend to look longer and more often at those whom they trust, respect, and care about than at those whom they dislike or mistrust. In some cultures, including the United States, direct eye contact conveys confidence and sincerity. Too little eye contact can indicate poor self esteem, while too much eye contact can indicate aggression and an attempt to control.

It is important to understand cultural differences regarding eye contact because not being aware of the norm in the new culture can lead to misconceptions. For example, the nurse who does not maintain eye contact during interactions often is considered untrustworthy, when, in fact, such eye contact actually may be considered rude and disrespectful in the nurse's native culture.

Physical Distance

Appropriate physical distance during communication and interactions can vary among cultures. In some cultures, acceptable personal and social distance is much closer than it is in the United States. Observe the distance your colleagues maintain when interacting among themselves, with patients and families, and with other health team members. Remember that appropriate physical distance is determined by the situation, the nature of the relationship, the topic under discussion, and your physical surroundings.

Touching

Touching, such as putting your arm around someone or putting your hand on another's arm or shoulder, can be used to convey caring, sympathy, encouragement, and praise—as well as anger, control, and restraint. It is very important to remember that the norms that govern touching behavior differ among cultures.

In the United States, a certain amount of distance usually is maintained when interacting with others, unless the situation requires close physical contact, for example, comforting a grieving patient or family member. If your culture is one in which touching or physical closeness is the norm, you may have to adjust your personal space to accommodate the norms of your new work environment.

Tone of Voice

When speaking, the tone of your voice can indicate a range of feelings and emotions, from calm approval to angry disapproval. Often it is not what is said, but *how* you say it, that can make a difference in the outcome of an interaction with a patient, colleague, or health team member. For example, when you are stressed or anxious, your voice often is high pitched or loud, and your words are spoken at a rapid pace. In this way, you transmit your stress to others. By taking a deep breath or two before speaking, and by consciously slowing your breathing, your voice will become lower pitched and calmer, the pace of your words will slow, and patients and colleagues will relax.

Time

The way in which we perceive and structure our time is also a form of nonverbal communication. Time perceptions include punctuality, willingness to wait, speed of speech, and how long people are willing to listen.

Time in the United States often is viewed as a commodity, and fairly rigid time constraints are practiced in the workplace. Arriving for work on time and leaving work on time are the expected norms—and U.S. labor laws require strict adherence to work hours. Being on time for meetings and appointments is seen as a matter of respect, and it is expected that patient care will be carried out quickly and efficiently and in an organized manner. The United States is considered a fast-paced culture. If the pace of your native culture is slower, you will have to be aware of the perception of time in the United States because you may have to adjust your pace accordingly.

All nurses should be aware of the messages they are sending with their nonverbal communication and should carefully observe the nonverbal cues that others may be sending—intentionally or unintentionally.

IDIOMS, SLANG, AND ABBREVIATIONS

Proficiency in communication also includes an understanding of the **idioms, jargon,** and **slang** of the new country and new work setting. Failure to understand may create a barrier to communication.

Idioms

An *idiom* is an expression of speech whose meaning is translated figuratively rather than literally. The meaning of an idiom is only known through common usage, thus idioms present a particular challenge for nurses entering a new culture—both a new host culture and a new employment culture. For example, in the United States you might hear a colleague say, "Well, I guess Mr. Jones will pull through." Translated, this means that Mr. Jones will recover—not that he will "pull" something. A patient may say to you, "I have to use the facilities." This means that he or she has to go to the bathroom or restroom.

Jargon

Jargon is a form of language used by people who work together within a specific occupation or profession or within a common interest group. It is a kind of shorthand for the group. For example, Digoxin is a common medication used in the United States. However, when nurses talk about the medication, they refer to it as "Dig" (using the first syllable of the word) rather than Digoxin as is seen in nursing textbooks.

Slang

Slang is the use of highly informal words or expressions that are not considered standard in the language. You will encounter slang expressions both in the workplace and in the community. For example, when you first meet someone, that person might say to you, "What's up?" or "How're you doing?" What the individual really is asking is, "How are you?"

A list of the common slang, jargon, and idioms used in the United States and identified in focus groups with foreign-educated nurses may be found in Appendix E.1. A list of slang terms, idioms, and jargon commonly heard in nursing practice situations may be found in Appendix E.2. Both appendices give the terms and phrases and their common meanings.

Communication Challenges

Lack of experience with such terms can result in misunderstandings and even errors. Foreign-educated nurses often find that other people's perception of them as competent professionals is directly related to their ability to speak English like a native. In focus groups conducted with CGFNS applicants (2000), one participant described her experience:

> Anybody coming to the U.S. needs American-spoken English because here they have their own way of speaking, so they need to understand spoken English the way it is spoken here. We like America obviously because we all moved here but it's just the way they treated us. I'm not saying we're better, but we are professionals and we just weren't treated as such.

Another focus group participant indicated that she had encountered a patient asking another nurse, "What did she say?" because the patient could not understand her accent and pronunciation. This nurse further indicated that such situations made her feel awkward and inadequate as a working professional. Another nurse confirmed this perspective by adding, "It is difficult to communicate with patients and doctors, even simple words, because of pronunciation."

Pronunciation, according to participants in the focus group, was considered a challenge—especially knowing what syllable to accent in a word—as was understanding the idioms and slang used not only in U.S. English but also as part of the language of nursing.

The focus group shared several examples of how idioms and slang (often substituted for universal clinical terms) had confused them, for example, the use of *puffer* for inhaler, when discussing asthma medication; *pickups* for forceps; *okie-dokie* for okay; *call the patient* or *pronounce the patient* for time of death; and the use of the terms *mad* (in some cultures a term for crazy) and *angry* interchangeably. In each of these examples, participants said that they had no idea what the slang terms meant when they first heard them. They felt they would have been better prepared for the workplace if they were more familiar with the idioms and slang commonly used in U.S. health care settings before they began nursing practice in the United States.

Abbreviations

Some participants in the focus group also reported difficulty reading charts and doctors' orders because of the various ways written English is used in the U.S. health care setting and because of the frequent use of abbreviations. In fact one nurse shared, "I read the chart and it said ABT, and I was embarrassed to ask what ABT means. But later I found that it means antibiotic treatment but I didn't know, and I felt bad. They use shortened forms for everything. Abbreviations are everywhere." A list of the abbreviations that focus group participants identified and their explanations may be found in Appendix E.3.

The use of abbreviations, however, is becoming less common in the United States. In an effort to promote patient safety, The Joint Commission reaffirmed its "Do Not Use" list of abbreviations in health care in May of 2005. The Do Not Use list identifies the abbreviations that can be misinterpreted and result in errors and that should not be used in the health care setting (see Figure 8.1). The Joint Commission is a nonprofit organization that evaluates and accredits over 15,000 health care organizations and programs in the United States, including hospitals, long-term care facilities and nursing homes, hospice services, and rehabilitation centers, to name a

Official "Do Not Use" List[1]

Do Not Use	Potential Problem	Use Instead
U (unit)	Mistaken for "0" (zero), the number "4" (four) or "cc"	Write "unit"
IU (International Unit)	Mistaken for IV (intravenous) or the number 10 (ten)	Write "International Unit"
Q.D., QD, q.d., qd (daily)	Mistaken for each other	Write "daily"
Q.O.D., QOD, q.o.d, qod (every other day)	Period after the Q mistaken for "I" and the "O" mistaken for "I"	Write "every other day"
Trailing zero (X.0 mg)* Lack of leading zero (.X mg)	Decimal point is missed	Write X mg Write 0.X mg
MS MSO4 and MgSO4	Can mean morphine sulfate or magnesium sulfate Confused for one another	Write "morphine sulfate" Write "magnesium sulfate"

[1] Applies to all orders and all medication-related documentation that is handwritten (including free-text computer entry) or on pre-printed forms.

*Exception: A "trailing zero" may be used only where required to demonstrate the level of precision of the value being reported, such as for laboratory results, imaging studies that report size of lesions, or catheter/tube sizes. It may not be used in medication orders or other medication-related documentation.

Additional Abbreviations, Acronyms and Symbols
(For possible future inclusion in the Official "Do Not Use" List)

Do Not Use	Potential Problem	Use Instead
> (greater than) < (less than)	Misinterpreted as the number "7" (seven) or the letter "L" Confused for one another	Write "greater than" Write "less than"
Abbreviations for drug names	Misinterpreted due to similar abbreviations for multiple drugs	Write drug names in full
Apothecary units	Unfamiliar to many practitioners Confused with metric units	Use metric units
@	Mistaken for the number "2" (two)	Write "at"
cc	Mistaken for U (units) when poorly written	Write "ml" or "milliliters"
µg	Mistaken for mg (milligrams) resulting in one thousand-fold overdose	Write "mcg" or "micrograms"

Figure 8.1. The "Do Not Use" list.

few. You can access The Joint Commission's Web site at http://www. jointcommission.org.

WHICH LANGUAGE TO USE

There have been reports of foreign-educated nurses regularly using their native, non-English language in the health care setting when there are coworkers from their home country also working on the unit. English-speaking nurses have complained about change-of-shift reports sometimes being in a language other than English, and patients have expressed dissatisfaction when nurses caring for them have engaged in conversations with each other in another language.

Some employers have reacted to these reports by going so far as to prohibit employees from speaking languages other than English in the workplace, even in staff lounges and cafeterias. Such reports have been cited by state policy makers as they seek to have English declared the official language of their state.

Acculturation Programs

Transition and **acculturation programs** for foreign-educated nurses generally support and reinforce the use of English in the workplace because it is necessary to ensure comprehensive and safe patient care. Employers are attempting to make both foreign- and U.S.-educated nurses who speak more than one language aware that non-English conversations around patients and coworkers who do not understand that language can be viewed as disrespectful. They are attempting to do this without minimizing the value of diversity in the U.S. workforce and the U.S. patient population.

It should be noted, however, that nurses from other countries bring not just ethnic and cultural diversity to the U.S. workforce, but also language diversity—and may be able to communicate with patients and families who do not speak English when other members of the health care team cannot do so.

Foreign-educated nurses report speaking such diverse languages as Spanish, French, Russian, Tagalog, Hindi, and Arabic, to name a few.

The most common non-English language used by foreign-educated nurses in practice in the United States is Spanish (CGFNS, 2002). Knowing the appropriate time to use a language other than English in the workplace is critical to being seen as a valuable member of the health care team.

SUMMARY

English language proficiency has been cited by nurse executives as critical to safe nursing care in the United States. As autonomous and accountable professionals, nurses are expected to advocate for their patients and to safely manage patient care. Proficiency in the English language, knowledge of the idioms and slang used in U.S. health care settings, assertiveness, good interpersonal skills, and being able to communicate effectively in the dominant language of the health care team are essential to accomplishing these roles.

As the U.S. population becomes more diversified, employers, government agencies, and businesses desire, and look for, professionals who are proficient in more than one language. The multilingual nurse is, and will continue to be, a valuable asset in the health care setting.

REFERENCES

The Commission on Graduates of Foreign Nursing Schools [CGFNS]. (2000). *Focus group report on the needs of foreign-educated nurses*. Unpublished report.

The Commission on Graduates of Foreign Nursing Schools [CGFNS]. (2002). *Characteristics of foreign nurse graduates in the United States workforce 2000–2001*. Philadelphia: Author.

U.S. Department of Health and Human Services, Office of Disease Prevention and Health Promotion. (2008). *Healthy People 2010*. Retrieved January 11, 2009, from http://www.health.gov/healthypeople/

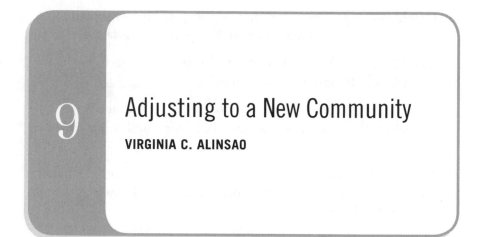

9 Adjusting to a New Community

VIRGINIA C. ALINSAO

In This Chapter

Housing

Transportation

Banking

Community Involvement

Safety

Summary

Keywords

Automated teller machines (ATMs): Street-side computerized devices that provide bank customers with access to their accounts and the ability to withdraw money from remote locations.

Check card purchase: Buying an item with a bank debit card that reduces the balance in your bank account.

Credit history: Record of an individual's past borrowing and repayment of money. Includes history of late payment and bankruptcy.

Credit rating: An estimate of somebody's ability to repay money given on credit based on credit history.

Credit union: Owned and controlled by its members, a cooperative bank association that provides loans and other financial services to its members.

Debit card: A plastic card that provides an alternative payment method to cash when making purchases; also known as a bank card *or* check card.

Default clause: Section in a document; part of a contract that explains the consequences if someone fails to pay a debt or to meet a financial obligation.

Direct deposit: Electronic delivery of a paycheck directly into an individual's bank account by the individual's employer.

Electronic transfer: Computer-based system used to perform financial transactions electronically.

Homeless shelter: Last resort in temporary housing for people in need who do not have a place to live.

Human resource department: Section of an organization responsible for coordinating the recruitment and hiring of employees as well as maintaining the organization's adherence to labor laws.

Identity theft: Theft of personal information, such as someone's bank account or credit card details.

Scam: A scheme for making money by dishonest means.

Security deposit: A sum of money required by somebody selling something or leasing property as security against the buyer's or tenant's failure to fulfill the contract.

Whether you have already arrived in the United States or are still planning your journey, this chapter provides useful information for making your initial stay as comfortable as possible. Some nurses plan to stay temporarily and others for long-term employment, but both will be in need of advice on how to manage within U.S. society. This chapter discusses several key topics that are useful for newly arriving nurse immigrants as they adjust to a new community in the United States.

HOUSING

No matter where you decide to settle in the United States, you will have many options for housing. The most common initial housing options available include: living with friends or family; renting a room in a house; sharing an apartment or house with coworkers or others; or renting an apartment by yourself or with your family. Some recruitment agencies or employers may coordinate housing arrangements for foreign-educated nurses, while others may not. If your housing is being selected for you prior to your arrival in the United States, you may wish to discuss housing options with the hiring agency and voice your preferences or requirements. If housing is not being selected for you, you should consider four factors when selecting housing: location, price, size, and privacy. If this is your first time living in the United States, it is a good idea to look for a residence convenient to your place of work, if possible.

To decide which housing option is best for you, ask yourself these questions:

- Do I prefer to live close to my place of work? Will I have a car, or will I rely on public transportation?
- How much of my income do I want to spend on housing costs? Are apartments near my place of work considerably more expensive than apartments in another part of the city?
- Do I have family members or friends who live in the same city, and do I prefer to live near them? Is there a community in this city where many other people from my country live, and do I prefer to live there?
- How much space do I need—or want—to live in? Am I coming to the United States with my family or alone? Will renting

a bedroom and sharing a bathroom and kitchen be sufficient, or do I need to rent a house to accommodate my family?

- Do I want to live alone or with others? Do I mind living with strangers, friends, or coworkers? Do I prefer to live in an apartment community or in a private residence?

Finding Housing

If you are responsible for finding your own housing, there are several ways in which to search. One popular way to search for housing—from abroad or within the United States—is by using a search engine. One widely used site is called "Craigslist." It is an easy-to-use online resource that lets you locate housing within any of the 50 states and U.S. territories. To use it, log on to http://www.craigslist.com and click on the state and city in which you wish to search for housing. Craigslist allows you to search for roommates, shared apartments, and rooms for rent, as well as private apartments that are either furnished or unfurnished. If this is your initial trip abroad, you can also use Craigslist to find new and used furniture, appliances, community services, events, and other valuable information. However, remember to limit the amount of personal information you provide online for safety purposes and to prevent **identity theft.** Always advise someone of your intended appointments or meetings with strangers met through Internet sites.

Other methods for finding housing or roommates include looking in the classifieds section of local newspapers (which may be available on the Web), searching online communities from your country of origin (e.g., http://www.sulekha.com for Indian nurses), looking on bulletin boards at local coffee shops or grocery stores, or asking your employer's **human resource department.** Often large hospitals have partnerships with apartment communities where discount rates may be available.

Renting an Accommodation

Selecting an apartment or house to rent is not always an easy task. Photos of accommodations placed online can be deceiving; it is always better to view housing in person. If you are not confident in your English-speaking skills, it is a good idea to take a friend with you when you go to look at the rental accommodation. Carefully examine all of the rooms, making sure that the appliances and utilities (stove, refrigerator, toilet, shower, lights, heat, and air conditioning) are working properly. In addition, it may be helpful to visit the neighborhood at night before making a decision about renting there.

If you rent a house or an apartment within a house, the property owner is commonly referred to as the *landlord,* and the renter is referred to as the *tenant.* If you rent an apartment that is part of an apartment building or community, you might not deal directly with the landlord; instead, you may be dealing with a property management company or an individual property manager. In some areas, the property manager may be known as the building superintendent, commonly referred to as the "super."

The Costs of Rentals

Rental costs vary and may depend on the residence's location, size, and amenities. Typically, it is cheaper to rent from a private landlord than from an apartment community because large communities offer amenities, such as swimming pools and fitness centers, which can increase the price of renting. In the United States, it is considered reasonable to spend about 25% of one's income on housing costs (U.S. Citizenship and Immigration Service, 2007), but in areas with especially high rents, such as New York City or San Francisco, it is often common for people to spend a higher percentage of their income on rent.

If utilities such as gas, electricity, and water are not included in the monthly fee, the renter will have to pay for these expenses separately each month. The cost of renting also depends on the duration of the rental period. It is usually less expensive to rent an apartment for 1 year than it is to rent for 3 months or on a month-to-month basis. Additionally, the time of year in which you move in may impact the price. Parts of the country experience seasonal high and low temperatures when people are less likely to move, and during these times rental companies offer lower rates to attract customers.

The Rental Process

Once you find and select a rental accommodation, there are several steps that may be required before you can move in. These steps include applying for occupancy, paying a **security deposit,** and signing a residential tenancy agreement (lease).

Laws regarding housing rentals vary greatly from state to state and sometimes vary even between cities in the same state. The information included here is general information only.

Rental Application. The first step in obtaining a rental accommodation is to fill out an application form. This form requires you to demonstrate your financial ability to pay the rent, which is usually based on your salary, your previous rental history, and your credit report. In addition, there also may be a criminal background check included. Many nurse migrants working in the United States for the first time will not have a rental or **credit history** and, therefore, will have to supply employment documentation and income verification. You will need to request such documents from your employer. Most property management companies require applicants to pay for the processing of the rental application; the application fee is usually $25 or $50. Always request receipts for money you have paid.

Security Deposit. Once you apply for a rental accommodation, the landlord or property manager may ask you to pay a security deposit. A security deposit is a sum of money you pay before moving in. It is typically the amount of 1 month's rent. Once the security deposit is paid, the landlord cannot rent the house or apartment to anyone else. The landlord keeps the security deposit in case you damage the property, fail to pay the rent, or leave without cleaning the rental properly. As long as you do no damage, pay the rent, and clean the rental after vacating it, you will receive your security deposit back after you move out. New immigrants may have to pay a security deposit in the amount of 2 or 3 months rent if they do not have a rental history or a credit history to show as proof of good financial standing.

Signing the Lease. A lease is a legal contract between the landlord/ property manager and the renter/tenant that outlines the responsibilities of each party. The lease states the rules and responsibilities of both parties and mainly includes the monthly rental price, the number of months the renter is required to pay, the date of the month the rent is due, the number of people allowed to reside in the unit, the number (if any) and size of pets allowed to reside in the unit, and specific property rules. Any repairs or changes to the property promised by the landlord or property manager also should be included in the lease.

Leases for the duration of 1 year are most common, but other lease options also exist, such as 3-, 6-, 9-, and 18-month terms. Month-to-month rental agreements also exist, but often for much higher rent.

The lease or rental agreement should also specify the number of days' notice required before moving out of the apartment. If your lease is scheduled to expire on December 31, for example, you may need to give 60 days notice to the landlord/property manager before vacating. In this case, you would need to specifically document, in writing, by October 31 that you wish to vacate the property on December 31.

Additionally, the lease will tell you the date by which you must pay your monthly rental fee. For example, the rent is normally due on the first of each month. However, the lease will usually specify a day (for example, the fifth of the month) by which the rent must be paid before late fees are assessed.

Terminating a Lease. Because the lease is a legally binding document, the renter is held by law to pay the entire term of the lease. However, there are ways to cancel—or "break"—a lease if you need to move out of the property before the contract has expired. Landlords will vary on the specific methods of breaking a lease. One example of a lease **default clause** is that the person responsible for renting the accommodation must pay 2 months rent if vacating the property prior to the expiration of the contract.

If you need to move out of the apartment immediately, you may ask permission from the landlord/property manager to *sublet* the apartment. Subletting allows you to rent your apartment to a third party for the duration of the lease.

Renter's Insurance

You may wish to purchase renter's insurance to protect the contents of your home—your furniture, clothing, books, and other possessions—against damage or theft. The cost of renter's insurance varies, but it usually averages $10 to $20 per month.

Paying for Utilities

Common utilities include water, electricity, natural gas, trash disposal, recycling, telephone, Internet, and cable television. In some apartments, the landlord will pay for water, electricity, and/or gas and will include these utilities in the monthly rental fee. Otherwise, tenants will pay for their own utilities. In this case, the landlord or management company usually will provide you with a list of service providers, which you must then call and ask to activate new service. Some utility companies may charge an activation fee for initiating the service. Others charge a small deposit fee, which you can pay by check, money order, or credit card. Most household bills and other transactions in the United States are paid for using one of these methods rather than cash (see section on banking in this chapter).

Household Appliances

Rental property almost always will be equipped with necessities, such as a cooking stove, an oven, and a refrigerator. Some apartments have electric stoves, while others use gas. Electric and gas stoves operate differently. If you are not familiar with how to operate the stove, ask the landlord or property manager for assistance.

Some rental properties come with additional kitchen equipment, such as a garbage disposal (located in the sink drain for shredding food waste), dishwasher, or microwave. Make sure the landlord or property manager shows you how to operate these appliances safely. For example, you need to know which switch turns the garbage disposal on and off; it can easily be confused with a light switch. *Never* stick your hand in the disposal while it is running. The disposal has sharp blades that can severely cut your hand and fingers. If you are unsure how to operate an appliance, ask the landlord to demonstrate its use.

Other appliances, such as a washing machine and clothes dryer, may not be included in your apartment. Many older apartment buildings have a common laundry facility that may require you to pay to use the washing machine and dryer. If no laundry facilities are available, then you may need to do your laundry at a public laundromat.

Furnished Versus Unfurnished Rentals

Your apartment may be rented as a "furnished" apartment—with living room, dining room, and bedroom furniture provided by the property owner—or as an "unfurnished" apartment. If the apartment is unfurnished, you will need to either rent or purchase the necessary furniture. If you are interested in renting furniture, there are companies that provide this service. If you are interested in purchasing furniture, you can either look for used furniture or buy new.

TRANSPORTATION

Public Transportation

Many, but not all, major cities in the United States provide public transportation services. The most common types of public transport are buses, subway, train, and streetcar services. Taxis are also common but cost more than public transportation.

City Buses

Public buses run along designated routes and have fixed stops to get on or off the vehicles. Bus schedules are available at bus stops, online, and in public libraries. Most bus systems require riders to pay the exact fare, meaning that you should always have change with you if you are riding the bus. Bus drivers generally cannot make change.

In some cities, you can buy daily, weekly, or monthly bus passes for frequent use.

Intercity Buses

Intercity buses provide transportation to the general public across U.S. cities and states. Intercity buses, also called coach buses, are generally less expensive than other commercial modes of transportation. A number of discount bus lines offering service along specific routes (New York to Washington, D.C.; New York to Boston; and, more recently, between some west coast cities) recently have grown in popularity. Schedules and fares can be viewed online, and tickets can be purchased either online or at the bus station.

Subway

The subway is an electronic, heavy rail service that provides frequent and rapid passenger transport in urban areas. The subway system can be operated either underground in tunnels or elevated above street level. The subway may be called various names depending on the city. Some, such as the New York subway, charge a flat fee per episode of travel. Other systems, such as the one in Washington, D.C., charge a fee based on the distance you travel.

Train

The United States has one of the lowest intercity rail usages in the developed world. Amtrak is the sole nationwide passenger rail carrier in the United States and offers regional train service throughout the country. Other companies offer regional rail service (particularly for commuters traveling from suburban areas into cities) in metropolitan areas around the country.

Streetcars

Streetcars are an electronic rail system used for urban public transportation. They function at the street level and, therefore, at a lower capacity and lower speed than a heavy rail metro system. Streetcars are sometimes also called trams, trolleys, or light rail.

Private Transportation

Air Travel

Travel by air is significantly more common in the United States than in some other parts of the world, largely due to the size of the country and the lack of widespread rail service. Flights in and out of major cities are frequent and can be found relatively easily. Depending on which part of the country you are flying out of, certain airline carriers are less expensive than others. Other factors, including the time of year and how far in advance you purchase your tickets, can have a significant impact on cost. There are many search engines that allow you to compare airfares and purchase tickets online. Another option is to use a travel agent when booking a flight or trip, but this option can be more costly.

Car Rental

Car rental is a common service in most U.S. cities, with a wide variety of companies in the industry. Some car rental agencies require you to have a major credit card to rent a vehicle, while others accept **debit cards** or cash deposits (see the banking section in this chapter). Most car rental agencies have minimum age requirements (typically between 18 and 25) for car renters.

Obtaining a Driver's License

If you plan to drive an automobile after moving to the United States, you must obtain a driver's license in the state in which you live. Information on how to obtain a license is available from your state's Department of Motor Vehicles (DMV). Even if you do not plan to drive, it is a good idea to get either a driver's license or a nondriver identification card from your state's DMV because these are commonly used forms of identification throughout the United States.

Motor vehicle laws and procedures will vary from state to state. Generally, to get a driver's license you will first need to apply for a Learner's Permit at the local DMV. In order to receive this permit, you will be required to take and pass a written examination on your state's traffic laws. In most states, a Driver's Handbook, containing a summary of the state's traffic laws, is available through the DMV. Following the test, you will take a driving test to obtain a driver's license.

BANKING

As soon as you arrive in the United States, you should open a bank account. For convenience, choose a bank with branches (offices) close to your work or home. Just as with any business transaction, banks have certain conditions on opening an account. You will need an acceptable form of identification—a valid passport or alien registration card, driver's license, or state identification card. Most banks also require a minimum deposit to open an account. Other financial institutions, such as **credit unions,** offer the same services as a commercial bank, but they are not-for-profit organizations that cater to specific groups of people, such as employees of a large university or state government. Ask your employer if they are affiliated with a credit union where you can become a member.

Insured Banks

Make sure that the bank you choose is insured by the Federal Deposit Insurance Corporation (FDIC). This is indicated by an FDIC decal at the front entrance of the bank. You also can check to see if a bank is FDIC-insured by going to http://www.fdic.gov. This is important because if an FDIC-insured bank closes its business for any reason, the federal government will reimburse the funds in your bank deposit accounts up to a maximum amount set by federal law. That amount is temporarily set at $250,000 until December 31, 2009, after which it will be $100,000. The National Credit Union Share Insurance Fund (NCUSIF) offers similar insurance for Credit Union deposits.

Checking and Savings Accounts

You should consider opening both a checking and a savings account at the bank you select. A savings account is for saving money for emergencies and large expenses, such as vacations, holiday gifts, or the down payment on a car. If you lose your job, for example, you can use the money you have saved to pay for rent, utilities, food, or transportation. The general advice is to have the equivalent of at least 3 months' salary in your savings account for unexpected expenses.

Use your checking account to pay your bills or to get cash from the bank. When you open a checking account, the bank will order you a booklet of checks that can be printed with your name and address. Before writing checks, make sure you have enough funds deposited in your checking account to cover the amount of the check that you write. An *overdraft* can occur if you do not have enough money to cover checks or withdrawals from your account. This a common mistake, and depending on the circumstances, the bank *may* or *may not* pay the check, **check card purchase,** or withdrawal; the bank will usually fine you an additional fee, sometimes daily, until you pay for the overdraft. However, intentionally *bouncing* (or writing bad checks) is a federal offense, and you can ruin your credit at stores and banks, in addition to possibly being fined, going to jail, or even being deported. In most cases, if you accidentally bounce a check and contact the payee as soon as you realize the error, they will allow you to pay them the value of the bounced check, along with any nominal service charges that may have resulted because of your mistake.

Monthly Statements

Each month, your bank will mail you a written statement or provide you with an online record showing you every transaction made in the previous month. Transactions include deposits, checks you wrote to others, cash withdrawals, earned interest, and any fees or penalties. Get in the habit of reviewing your bank statement as soon as you receive it. If you find an error in the statement, there are written instructions on the back of the document telling you what you should do to report it. It is important to follow these instructions carefully because there is a time limit for filing such complaints.

Depositing Funds

The most convenient way to deposit or to withdraw cash from your account is through one of your bank's **automated teller machines** (ATMs). ATMs can usually be found throughout the area in a number of different locations. Your bank will issue you an ATM card at the time you open your account. The bank can also issue a debit card, which can be used both as an ATM card and to make purchases, but you must ask for it. At that time, you will be asked to provide a 4-digit number, called a personal identification number (PIN), which is necessary to use the card. Make sure it is a memorable number, and *never* share it with anyone. Be aware that if you use your ATM card to withdraw money from an ATM belonging to an institution other than your bank, you may have to pay an additional service charge for each transaction.

Direct Deposit

To avoid having to go to the bank or ATM to deposit each paycheck, you can authorize your employer to use a transaction called **direct deposit.** As the term implies, on paydays your paycheck automatically is deposited electronically into your account. You can designate a portion of your paycheck to be deposited to your checking account and a portion to your savings account.

Electronic Banking

Another convenient way to do your banking is electronically through online banking. Using the Internet, you can visit your bank's personal and secure Web site to check your account information and **electronically transfer** funds. Beware of **scams,** however. Never share your banking information online, on the telephone, or though the mail without using great caution. If you have any questions or doubts about e-mails, telephone calls, or mailings that ask you for personal banking information, call your bank directly and confirm.

Remittances

At some point, you may wish to send money back to your home country. Family and friends may refer you to one of several overseas money wiring services, but be sure to ask about fees for this service and the safeguards that will protect your money. Make sure that you know exactly when the recipient will retrieve the funds in either local currency or in U.S. dollars, and don't forget to check with your local bank, which may offer a similar service at a lower cost.

Credit Cards

Many U.S. residents use credit cards to purchase items or services. This is a convenient way to pay for goods and services when you may not have cash with you or sufficient funds in your checking account on a particular day. However, it is also an easy way to acquire significant debt.

Credit Card Payments

Failing to pay your credit card bill completely at the end of a billing cycle will result in interest charges on the amount you still owe. Make sure you understand the terms and interest rate of your credit card, as they vary widely. All credit card companies assess a finance charge for late payment or if you exceed your credit limit. The credit card company may also increase your interest rate for late payment.

Always pay at least the minimum amount or more (preferably the full balance) by the due date on the statement you receive from the credit card company. It is good practice to mail your payment at least a week before the due date to avoid a late payment. Online payments, if made by a certain time, usually are credited the same day.

Credit History

Your interest rate may be higher on your credit card if you do not have a credit history in the United States. One way to prove your credit worthiness is to provide a copy of your job offer letter with salary information and the length of the contract. Most banks honor this documentation and may issue a credit card with a lower credit limit.

In the United States, a good credit history is essential. You can usually get a good **credit rating** if you pay all of your bills on time and keep your balances (how much you owe) low. In addition to paying your credit card bills on time, you should pay your gas and electric bill, landline and mobile telephone service, cable service, rent or mortgage, and car payments on time. Keep your credit card balances low or at zero, and do not apply for too many loans and credit cards. A good credit rating will make it easier to get a lower credit card interest rate and obtain a loan for a car or a home with a favorable interest rate.

Credit Card Security

Carry your credit cards in a safe place to avoid misplacing them or having them stolen. Write down your credit card numbers and the company contact information, and keep it separate from your credit cards. This way, if you lose your wallet with your credit cards in it, you can immediately report the loss to the credit card company and cancel your credit cards. In most cases, you will not be responsible for fraudulent charges if you notify the company right away.

COMMUNITY INVOLVEMENT

Getting involved in your new community may be hard at first, but making the effort to get to know your neighbors will help you feel more connected to your community and better able to enjoy your new life in the United States. Simple gestures, such as introducing yourself and greeting your neighbors whenever you see them, are a good start.

Community Organizations

Visit the city or town hall in your community to inquire about community organizations and recreational activities that you and your family can join, or volunteer for projects that benefit your community. When you arrive in the United States, you should visit your home country's consulate or embassy. This office also can provide information about various hometown associations and volunteer projects. Informal immigrant organizations, known as *Hometown Associations* (HTA), also can play a critical role in an immigrant's integration into the community. HTAs offer support services such as language classes, day care, and resources to other community services.

Government Services

Most U.S. state governments have offices for "New Americans" that offer services for recent immigrants. There also are nongovernmental organizations (NGOs), such as the Foreign Born Information and Referral Network (FIRN; http://www.firnon-line.org), that work to ensure equal access to community resources and opportunities for all foreign-born individuals. These organizations welcome volunteers.

Religious Organizations

Other ways to get involved in your new community is through your place of worship, the schools your children attend, or through your work. Your place of worship may initiate a special project for the poor, or provide opportunities for members to volunteer at a **homeless shelter.** Your child's school may need volunteers to accompany students on school trips or participate in Parent–Teacher Association (PTA) activities. At work, your coworkers may ask you to volunteer or donate to a special community project.

Public Libraries

Finally, the public library is open to everyone and provides mostly free and valuable resources and library staff that can help you. The public library is also a great place to review materials and literature about events happening in your community. There are many opportunities for community involvement. You can do your part and feel connected to your new community by participating in local, state, and national projects and initiatives.

SAFETY

From popular television programs, newspapers, magazines, and the Internet, you may already have an impression of safety issues in the United States. Sometimes the reality can be quite different from what is magnified through the media, but being in a new and different culture, far from family and friends, can foster a sense of vulnerability and helplessness. Unfortunately, immigrants can be easy targets for dishonest individuals. Criminals may take advantage of them because immigrants may be less likely to report a crime.

Law Enforcement Agencies

Law enforcement agencies in the United States exist to protect all members of a community from harm. If you come in contact with a police officer, there are certain things that you should know. When an officer approaches you, you should be polite and cooperative. If an officer stops you while driving, immediately pull your vehicle to the side of the road and stop. When the officer approaches you, do not make any sudden movements. Do not reach for your identification until the officer instructs you to do so. Additionally, do not get out of the car unless the police officer instructs you to do so. Keep your hands where the officer can see them, and do not attempt to reach into your pockets or other areas of the car. *Never* attempt to bribe a police officer, as this is a crime in the United States. You can ask the officer to show you his or her identification and badge.

Emergency Systems

Emergencies do happen, and everyone must plan for them. In the United States, the emergency number is 911. You can call this number from any landline or mobile telephone. Only call 911 for life-threatening medical emergencies, to report a fire, or to report a crime in progress or suspicious activities, such as screams or calls for help.

All 911 calls are recorded, and operators are trained to handle emergencies. Nonemergency phone numbers can be found by looking in your local telephone book.

When you call 911, stay calm. Remember your location (your home address or present location), and be prepared to describe the emergency. Do not hang up until you have answered all the questions posed by the operator. If you do not speak English well, let the operator know. This is the time to practice one basic sentence: "I do not speak English well. I speak [Cantonese or Vietnamese, etc.]." The operator will get an interpreter on the line to help you communicate.

Also, become acquainted with the police department near your house or apartment. Keep the telephone numbers of your local emergency service providers visible and accessible at all times in your home. That includes the police department, the fire and emergency rescue department, the poison control center, as well as the local animal control office.

SUMMARY

Generally, the concerns of foreign-educated nurses when they first come to the United States are about housing, transportation, and personal safety. Addressing these concerns as early as possible in the immigration process will help you to adapt more quickly to a new country and a new work environment.

There are many resources available to everyone in the United States. Our citizens welcome and value the contribution of all international workers. We realize that all people add to the tapestry of this great land of opportunity!

Preparation is one key to your success as a new resident of the United States. By knowing what to expect when you arrive, you will spend less time wondering and worrying and more time enjoying your new life and community.

RESOURCES

Foner, N., & Alba, R. (2006). *The second generation from the last great wave of immigration: Setting the record straight. Migration Policy Institute.* Retrieved October 6, 2008, from http://www.immigrationinformation.org/issue_Oct06.cfm

Hopkins Medicine. http://www.hopkinsmedicine.org/security/CS/crimeprev.htm

Maryland Department of Transportation. http://www.sha.state.md.us/safety

Migration Policy Institute. (2008). *Hometown associations: An untapped resource for immigrant integration?* Retrieved October 31, 2008, from http://migrationpolicy.org/news/2008_07_15.php

REFERENCE

U.S. Citizenship and Immigration Service. (2007). *Welcome to the United States. A Guide for New Immigrants.* Retrieved October 17, 2008, from http://www.uscis.gov/portal/site/uscis

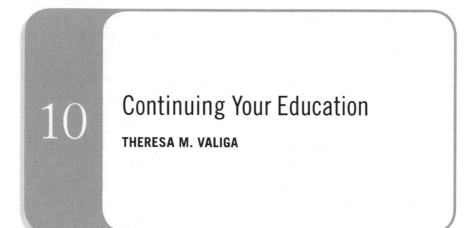

10 Continuing Your Education

THERESA M. VALIGA

In This Chapter

Improvements in Nursing Education

Higher Education in the United States

Educational Options in Nursing

Getting Information on Educational Options

Applying to Schools

Getting the Most Out of Your Education in the United States

Student Rights and Responsibilities

Summary

Keywords

Licensed practical nurse: A technical nurse with 12–18 months of training who has passed the state licensure examination for practical nurses (NCLEX-PN) and who works under the supervision of a registered nurse.

Public policy expert: An individual who has studied and/or works in the branch of political science that deals with the formation of laws or policies.

Registered nurse: A professional nurse with 2–4 years of education who has passed the state licensure examination for registered nurses (NCLEX-RN).

Translational scientists: Scholars who integrate research inputs from the basic sciences, social sciences, and political sciences to optimize both patient care and also preventive measures that may go beyond the provision of health care services.

Tuition reimbursement: Employer payment for a course of study. The employer may pay for the course before it starts or pay back course fees paid by the employee after completion of the course and attainment of a passing grade.

Nursing in the United States has undergone tremendous changes in recent years, and the profession continues to create new opportunities and options for educational preparation and advancement. This chapter focuses on the types of nursing education programs in the United States, the requirements for entry, students' rights and responsibilities, and nonacademic continuing education.

IMPROVEMENTS IN NURSING EDUCATION

Nurses who provide patient care and those who teach in schools of nursing are better prepared educationally than ever before. The science that provides the foundation for nursing practice is increasingly being built through the scholarly efforts of nurses. Collaborative partnerships between nurses and other health care professionals continue to evolve. In addition, the opportunities for nurses to influence the health of people through roles such as nurse practitioners, nurse midwives, home care clinicians, managers and administrators, health educators, acute and long-term care clinicians, researchers, and faculty are growing dramatically.

In order to prepare nurses for basic and advanced levels of practice, educational programs also have undergone tremendous changes in recent years. Curricula are increasingly creative and interactive, rather than rigid. Education is more learner-focused than teacher-centered. Clinical experiences for students reflect a greater emphasis on community-based care, health promotion, disease prevention, family involvement, and patient self-care. And nursing education programs are increasingly integrating technology and using distance learning strategies.

Nursing education programs are placing increased emphasis on documenting their outcomes and demonstrating that their graduates do, indeed, have the patient care, critical thinking, and communication abilities needed to function in the complex, constantly changing U.S. health care system. Finally, nurse educators are realizing that teaching nursing is both an art and a science—just as practicing nursing is an art and a science—and they are seeking greater preparation in curriculum development and evaluation, creative teaching/learning strategies, student and program evaluation, and other areas that complement their clinical specialty and expertise.

HIGHER EDUCATION IN THE UNITED STATES

Despite these exciting changes, higher education in the United States remains essentially unchanged from the structure established long ago. Generally, students must complete a high school (secondary school) education in order to be admitted to a college or technical school.

Technical schools may be independent, for-profit organizations, or they may be part of a community's high school. The focus of programs in such schools is more practical in nature. Some practical nurse programs are located in technical schools, and in some instances, students complete these program requirements while simultaneously completing their high school requirements.

For the majority of higher education in the United States, however, students complete their high school requirements and then apply for admission to a junior, community, or 2-year college; a liberal arts or comprehensive 4-year college or university; or a senior university. Individuals also may (and often do) apply for admission to such schools as adults, after having worked, completed military service, or raised a family. In fact, more and more students are beginning their college education as experienced adults, rather than immediately after high school, and the average age of enrolled students in many schools (particularly community colleges) is increasing.

Community Colleges

A community college (also known as a junior college) is a publicly supported institution that typically offers a wide range of courses and areas of study at reasonable costs. On a full-time basis, students would ordinarily complete such a program in 2 years, but because community colleges enroll many adult learners who work and raise families while going to school, it may take as long as 10 years for individuals to complete the program, which typically requires 60 credits. Upon completion of such a program, the individual will be awarded an associate degree in the area of study.

Liberal Arts Colleges

A liberal arts or 4-year college often offers courses only at the undergraduate (or baccalaureate) level, though some also offer master's programs. The primary emphasis in such schools is on providing a sound, comprehensive liberal arts education, and teaching and learning are highly important in such environments. Often the ratio of students to teachers is small, and individualized learning is valued. Upon completion of a program in such a school—which typically requires 120 credits and would be completed in 4 years on a full-time basis—students are awarded a Bachelor of Arts (BA) or Bachelor of Science (BS) degree.

Liberal arts colleges often are private, meaning that they receive little or no support from local or state governments; consequently, the tuition is higher than at public institutions. In response to the increased cost, however, many of these schools are able to offer students financial aid to support their enrollment.

Post-Graduate Focus

Individuals also may earn a BA or BS degree in a comprehensive university, which, in addition to a wide range of undergraduate programs, also offers a number of master's programs. Historically, comprehensive universities did not offer doctoral education, but that is changing in light of the growing need for individuals with such preparation in so many fields.

Again, a strong liberal arts foundation is valued in such institutions, but there may be more of an emphasis on research, science, and professional education than is often the case in a liberal arts college. Often, comprehensive universities are larger than liberal arts colleges, and there is greater diversity among the faculty and students. They may be public or private, and their tuition spans the range of reasonable to costly.

Senior Universities

Senior universities often are quite large (some with as many as 50,000 students enrolled), may be public or private, and may incorporate health science centers. They typically offer a wide range of baccalaureate, master's, and doctoral programs, and while teaching is an important part of the mission of such universities, faculty often are engaged extensively in research and practice activities. Tuition at public or state-owned senior universities typically is more reasonable than that of private schools.

Standard U.S. Requirements for Completion

Regardless of the type of institution in which the program is offered, a baccalaureate program in the United States usually requires 120 credits, a master's program requires anywhere between 30 and 60 post-baccalaureate credits, and a doctoral program may require an additional 30 or more post-master's credits. The usual progression of study has been to complete the baccalaureate degree, then proceed to the master's level and, finally, to the doctorate. However, in some fields (e.g., chemistry) students progress from a bachelor's degree to the doctoral program without earning a master's degree on the way, and in other fields (e.g., art), the master's is considered the terminal or final degree available.

In light of this complex and constantly changing higher education environment, the structure and options for preparation as a nurse have changed in recent years. Additional innovations in nursing education are expected as the need for, and value of, student-centered learning becomes increasingly evident; as life circumstances challenge the traditional full-time program option; as educational research informs faculty of the effectiveness of various models of teaching and learning, and as the profession evolves.

EDUCATIONAL OPTIONS IN NURSING

Initial and ongoing preparation for nursing roles is varied and complex. Education to be a **licensed practical nurse** (LPN) is generally 12 to 18 months in length and provided in vocational programs. Graduates of these programs are eligible to sit for the practical nurse licensure examination (the NCLEX-PN). LPNs (who are known as licensed vocational nurses [LVNs] in California and Texas) generally function under the supervision of a **registered nurse** (RN).

Initially, individuals can prepare for the RN role through one of three kinds of programs: (a) a 2-year associate degree program, typically located in a community college or junior college; (b) a 3-year, hospital-based program (referred to as a diploma program); or (c) a 4-year baccalaureate program offered through a college or university. Graduates of all three types of programs take the same examination for RN licensure (the NCLEX-RN), and all are prepared for beginning practice as a generalist nurse.

Articulation Programs

Licensed practical nurses who desire to become RNs often do so by enrolling in an associate degree program, and RNs who received their initial nursing education in an associate degree (ADN) or diploma program often decide to return to school to earn a baccalaureate degree in nursing (BSN). Many schools have designed programs especially for these RN students and refer to them as RN-to-BSN, ADN-to-BSN, or BSN-completion programs.

The programs generally eliminate repetition of content that RN students have already learned and build upon students' prior clinical experiences. RN-to-BSN programs typically are offered on a part-time basis and often during evenings or on weekends in order to accommodate nurses' work schedules. These programs remain focused on the preparation of a generalist nurse, not a nurse specialist.

Master's Education in Nursing

In the United States, nursing specialization is achieved at the graduate level, generally in master's degree programs. The master's degree one earns in nursing may be known as a Master of Science in Nursing (MSN), a Master of Science (MS), or a Master of Nursing (MN) degree. There also is one program in the country that awards the Master of Science in Nursing Education (MEd).

Most master's programs in nursing currently require completion of the baccalaureate degree for admission, but more and more schools are creating programs (e.g., RN-to-MSN) that allow RNs with an associate degree to be admitted directly to the master's program. Prior to enrolling in the clinical nursing courses in these programs, students must take courses and demonstrate that they have met baccalaureate-level competencies, but they are not required to complete every baccalaureate degree requirement (e.g., history), nor do they earn a bachelor's degree. They are awarded a master's degree upon completion of the entire program.

Master's programs are offered on either a full-time or part-time basis, and they are designed to prepare students for a particular specialty area of practice. Students may prepare for an advanced clinical practice role as a nurse practitioner, nurse midwife, clinical nurse specialist, or nurse anesthetist. They also may prepare for an advanced role as a nurse educator, nurse administrator, or another nurse specialist role that requires advanced education. Master's programs generally require 1 or 2 years of full-time study and integrate a core of advanced knowledge (e.g., research, leadership) with advanced knowledge related to specialty practice (e.g., functioning as a family nurse practitioner). See chapter 7 for additional information on advanced practice nursing.

Post-Master's Certificate in Nursing

The nurse's role in today's health care environment requires that individuals continually learn and grow professionally. In addition, the varied career opportunities available to nurses often lead some to consider pursuing a new role. Individuals who already hold a master's degree may return to school to complete a post-master's certificate program. These programs often are 12–15 credits in length and require students to enroll only in the specialty courses needed to prepare them for the new role. For example, a clinical nurse specialist who decides to pursue a career as an educator in an academic setting may enroll in a post-master's certificate program to take courses in principles of learning, curriculum development, integration of technology into education, program evaluation, test construction, and implementation of the faculty role.

Post-master's certificate programs award academic credit, and they present a certificate to those who complete the program. However, students are not awarded a degree for completion of such a program.

Doctoral Education for Nurses

Many nurses who hold master's degrees choose to return to school for a doctoral degree. Doctoral programs in nursing can be clinically based or research focused. The Doctor of Nursing Practice (DNP) degree is a new option in graduate nursing education, and its focus is still being clarified.

Preparation of Translational Scientists

For the most part, DNP programs are focused on advancing clinical nursing practice. They are designed to provide graduates with the skills and tools necessary to assess the evidence gained through nursing research, to evaluate the impact of that research on nursing practice, and to lead changes in health care based on that research—in order to enhance the quality of care provided to patients, families, and communities. Graduates of DNP programs, then, may be thought of as **translational scientists** rather than research scientists because they translate research into practice.

Preparation of Research Scientists

Research scientists, on the other hand, are prepared through Doctor of Philosophy (PhD) or Doctor of Nursing Science (DNSc/DNS/DSN) programs (or the one EdD in nursing education program available in the United States). In such programs there is a heavy emphasis on research methods, the conduct of research, data analysis, and the dissemination of research findings to appropriate audiences.

Course work may be individualized to meet students' learning and scholarship needs. Because many of their graduates pursue faculty roles, these programs often include learning experiences that help prepare students for an academic career.

Innovative Programs

In recent years, many nursing schools have developed innovative programs that allow nurses with diplomas or associate degrees to earn combined baccalaureate and graduate degrees. These include BSN-to-PhD, RN-to-DNP, and RN-to-PhD programs. The number of these innovative programs is increasing, and it is expected that this will continue to occur.

Once students enrolled in BSN-to-PhD, RN-to-DNP, or RN-to-PhD programs have achieved their baccalaureate-level competencies, they go on to enroll in graduate-level courses to begin preparation for their specialty. In many such programs, students take baccalaureate-level and graduate courses concurrently, or graduate-level courses are substituted for undergraduate-level requirements.

In addition to pursuing a doctoral degree in nursing, nurses sometimes choose to pursue a doctorate in another field (e.g., education, psychology, physiology), if such a program is closely aligned with their professional goals. Thus, one cannot assume that a nurse who uses the credential PhD after his/her name holds that degree in nursing. One can be assured, however, that the individual has completed a rigorous program that has prepared him/her to think and act differently.

Leadership Roles

It is expected that all nurses who hold master's or doctoral degrees will provide leadership within the profession and within the health care system. Their specialized preparation as clinicians, educators, administrators, **public policy experts,** translational scientists, or research scholars enables them to develop a vision for the future of nursing and enables them to engage colleagues to work toward realizing that vision. Their specialized preparation also enables them to study the impact of change on patient care, education, public policy, and the overall health of the nation.

Distance and Online Education

Distance or online education is different from traditional education in that classes are taken from a person's home rather than attending classes at a college, school, or university. Online education, rather than distance education, is the preferred term to use in describing this form of educational program. Online education involves providing classes and courses using Web-based programs and the Internet. Online educational programs can lead to a degree or a certificate indicating special knowledge, or they can provide continuing education for professional development. It is recommended, however, that you check the validity of all online programs with the State Board of Nursing and the Better Business Bureau. Some programs may not be authentic and may be considered "diploma mills."

How Do Online Programs in Nursing Education Work?

Several institutions of higher education offer online programs. These programs are accredited by university and nursing accrediting bodies and offer financial aid. Schools also offer tuition assistant programs, and the federal government offers assistance in the form of loans and grants. See Appendix F for a select listing of schools offering online nursing degrees.

Online nursing education programs vary from school to school and are generally hosted on the school's own Web site. The instructors for particular classes post lecture materials and assignments to the site, and there is usually a bulletin board or other discussion forum where students may post comments and questions. Assignments are e-mailed to the instructor usually on designated due dates. For many online classes, written course work takes the place of traditional examinations.

In these online courses, generally, the nonclinical component of the coursework is done online. Because there are no schools that allow nurses to fulfill the clinical requirements online, the clinical requirements are usually arranged at a medical facility near the individual's home.

While some online classes or degree programs allow students to complete course work at their own pace, many programs affiliated with traditional universities require online students to maintain the same quarter or semester schedule as on-campus students. Many online classes are structured around a series of assignments and examinations, and online course content generally is the same as that of traditional courses.

What Nursing Degrees Are Most Commonly Offered Online?

There are online programs for LPN-to-RN, RN-to-BSN, BSN-to-MSN, MSN-to-PhD, and MSN programs. However, the RN-to-BSN and MSN degrees are the most commonly offered online degrees. Although some institutions offer a variety of advanced degrees, there are also certificate options for students seeking certification in specialized areas of nursing practice.

What Prerequisites Are Required for Online Nursing Degrees?

There are prerequisites for online nursing degrees, and you should check with the school you are interested in to learn about the specific entrance requirements of the degree program. In general, BSN programs, whether online or traditional, have the following requirements:

- SAT or ACT exam, minimum scores vary widely by school
- Minimum GPA's range from 2.0 to 3.25, depending on the school
- 3 years of high school math, including geometry and algebra 2
- 3 years of high school science, including biology and chemistry
- 4 years of high school English
- 2 years of high school foreign language

RN-to-BSN, RN-to-MSN, and MSN programs generally require the following:

- Graduation from a nursing school that is accredited by either the National League for Nursing Accrediting Commission (NLNAC) or the Commission on Collegiate Nursing Education (CCNE)
- A current RN nursing license
- A 2.5 to 3.0 grade point average (GPA) in selected prerequisite courses

Other certificate programs have their own specific prerequisites, and schools generally list these in their catalogs or on their Web site. These online degree and certificate programs are designed for nurses at all levels who want to expand their skills and qualifications, pursue specialized areas of practice, or advance into supervisory or teaching roles.

Registered nurses with an associate degree or diploma certificate can build on their education and experience to earn a Bachelor of Science in Nursing (BSN). RNs without a formal nursing degree may also qualify to enter programs leading to a BSN or MSN. There are also master's programs in specialties, such as health care education.

What Are the Costs of Online Nursing Education Programs?

Costs of online nursing education offerings vary widely by school and degree program. Applicants should check the school's Web site for tuition and fees. Students enrolled in online degree programs are eligible for the same types of scholarships and financial aid as students enrolled in traditional programs.

There are many grants, loans, scholarships, work-study, and loan forgiveness programs available for qualifying candidates. The financial aid office at the school to which you apply can assist you with this information.

Also, many workplaces offer **tuition reimbursement** for both online and traditional nursing programs. This reimbursement may cover all or part of the cost of your courses. Generally, the employee must remain with that employer for at least 180 days following completion of the final course. You should check with your employer to see if tuition reimbursement is offered.

What Type of Computer Equipment Is Needed?

The computer equipment needed varies from program to program, but students planning to enroll in online classes should expect to have regular access to a computer with an Internet connection and a personal e-mail account. Schools will identify their specific requirements.

In summary, an increasing demand for nurses of all skill levels makes the accessibility and convenience of online nursing education a suitable choice to advance one's education. A select list of schools that provide online degree programs can be found at: http://www. earnmydegree.com/on-line-education/nursing.

Continuing Education in Nursing

Another route to continuing one's education is through more informal programs that may be offered outside the college or university setting and that typically do not award academic credit. Continuing education (CE) courses often are short, focused, and time-limited. They may take the form of a half-day workshop, a 1-hour online program, or a week-long intensive experience. They may be offered by academic institutions, professional organizations, health care centers, or independent CE businesses, and they are available in classroom, clinical or laboratory, video or online/distance formats, and in professional publications. CE credit is awarded upon successful completion of such learning experiences, and while such credits will not earn the individual an academic degree, they may be required to maintain one's license as an RN or LPN/LVN and to demonstrate continued competence in nursing.

GETTING INFORMATION ON EDUCATIONAL OPTIONS

There are many educational options available to foreign-educated nurses who wish to continue their education after they begin working in the United States. With so many choices available, however, it may be difficult to find information about various programs and make decisions about a course of advancement. However, in this age of technology, there are many ways to get information about education options and about specific nursing schools.

Organizational Resources

Among the most comprehensive resources available are two national nursing organizations: the National League for Nursing (NLN) and the American Association of Colleges of Nursing (AACN). The NLN (http://www.nln.org) publishes information annually about practical nurse programs, all prelicensure RN programs (i.e., associate degree, diploma, and baccalaureate), and graduate programs. The AACN (http://www.aacn.nche.edu/) publishes information annually about baccalaureate and graduate programs. Through these resources, potential students can learn the name, location, and types of programs offered at the more than 1,500 schools of nursing in the United States.

Another source of information about schools of nursing are the profession's two academic accrediting bodies—the National League for Nursing Accrediting Commission (NLNAC) (http://www.nlnac. org) and the Commission on Collegiate Nursing Education (CCNE) (http://www.aacn.nche.edu/Accreditation/). In the United States, program accreditation is voluntary, but most nursing programs pursue it. Accreditation of a program indicates that it has undergone rigorous peer review and has been determined to meet criteria for quality nursing education. Thus, a program's accreditation status is an important consideration for potential students.

Internet Resources

Information about nursing schools also may be found through various Web sites including:

- All Nursing Schools (http://www.allnursingschools.com)
- Discover Nursing (http://www.discovernursing.com)
- National Student Nurses Association (NSNA; http://www.nsna. org/)
- Nurses for a Healthier Tomorrow (http://www.nursesource. org/nursing_careers.html)

Journals and Magazines

In addition, magazines such as *U.S. News & World Report* regularly publish reports about academic institutions. They may rank graduate programs, or describe schools that offer quality education at a low price, or outline the "best" programs in a particular field. While such reports and rankings are helpful, one must use caution when reading them to examine the basis for the rankings.

For example, schools often are ranked based on the amount of funding they receive from the Federal government to support research activities. Or they may be ranked highly because many of their faculty are doctorally prepared or because their alumni give generously to the school. While criteria such as these may be important, one must be aware that they are not measures of the quality of education a student receives, the nature of student–teacher relationships that exist, or the innovativeness and effectiveness of the programs offered.

State Regulatory Boards

Finally, the Board of Nursing in each state and U.S. territory provides information about the practical nurse, prelicensure RN, advanced practice, and specialty graduate programs offered in that state. You can search the Web for "Board of Nursing" and then the specific state—or enter the Web site of the National Council of State Boards of Nursing (http://www.ncsbn.org) and click on the link to the specific state board.

APPLYING TO SCHOOLS

All nurses considering advancing their education are encouraged to contact or visit nursing schools to discuss the programs they offer and how those offerings can help meet their professional goals. In fact, such exploration is essential before applying to ensure that there is a good match between the program and your goals.

When considering studying nursing at the undergraduate, master's, or doctoral level, candidates need to look carefully at a number of factors, including costs, financial aid, admission requirements, length of program, graduation requirements, and employment opportunities. Although this is not intended to be a complete list, the following questions are important to consider when selecting a program:

- What courses in and outside nursing are required of students in the program? Will they help you build the knowledge base and the skills you need to pursue your professional career?
- How much flexibility is there in the program? Are there opportunities to select courses that are of interest to you? Are there opportunities to design individualized learning experiences

(e.g., clinical experiences, the topic of a course paper, the case studies you develop) that will meet your own needs?

- What kinds of clinical experiences are available for students? Will you be able to work with diverse populations and in a variety of settings (e.g., acute care hospitals, home care agencies, hospice settings, clinics, community health centers, etc.)? What role do students have in selecting their clinical experiences?
- What are the qualifications of the faculty? Are they prepared at the master's or doctoral level in nursing (or in the nursing-related specialty they teach, such as pharmacology)? Do they maintain a clinical practice? Are they scholars in their areas of teaching? Are they leaders in their field?
- What technology is available to support students in the program? Are the library, practice laboratories, and computer centers comprehensive and current, offering state-of-the-art technology and technological support?
- What resources are available to support students in the program? Are there advisors who are sensitive to the needs of students and able to help them be successful in the program? Is there a financial aid counselor in the school of nursing to explain special financial options available to nursing students? Is the school a recipient of a state or federal grant award?
- What are the relationships like among students and between students and faculty? Is there a spirit of learning together? Do students have the opportunity to work collaboratively on projects? Are master's and doctoral students able to work with faculty on the faculty member's research? Do faculty see themselves as learners as well as teachers?
- Is the program accredited by the NLNAC or CCNE?

While location and cost may be relevant when considering schools, asking questions such as these will help you apply to the school or schools that best fit your educational needs and career goals—not just the school that is closest or least expensive. Education is a critical investment, and it is important that the program in which you enroll will provide excellent learning experiences and prepare you for the roles you wish to pursue throughout your nursing career.

Admission Requirements

You should also be aware of each school's admission requirements. Students who are not native to the United States often are required to take the TOEFL (Test of English as a Foreign Language) and score at or above a level determined by each school. Admission to associate degree and baccalaureate programs usually requires achievement of a predetermined score on a standardized admission test, such as the SAT (http://www.collegeboard.com/student/testing/sat/about.html) or the ACT (http://www.act.org/aap/), as well as completion of specified high school courses (e.g., biology, chemistry) or specified prerequisites (e.g., anatomy and physiology, developmental psychology).

Admission to a master's program usually requires attainment of a predetermined score on the Graduate Record Exam (GRE), which is a standardized test of verbal, mathematics, and writing skills (http://www.ets.org/gre/), and completion of specified degrees (e.g., BSN) and courses (e.g., statistics). Admission to a doctoral program often requires the GRE, high academic achievement in previous courses, a writing sample, and formulation of a proposed area of research.

All schools have faculty or staff available to help potential students understand the admission requirements and processes, and you are encouraged to use those resources to be successful.

GETTING THE MOST OUT OF YOUR EDUCATION IN THE UNITED STATES

Foreign-educated nurses who continue their study of nursing after they enter the United States should expect to find undergraduate and graduate programs that are challenging, innovative, and designed to meet their individual needs as learners. The program should be learner-focused, with students actively involved in the learning process.

You should expect state-of-the-art practice laboratories that will help you learn and enhance a variety of skills including comprehensive assessment, decision making, team collaboration, and technological skills. You should expect to find library, information, and technology services that will allow you to access the broadest possible resources, to be creative in teaching patients about managing their own health, to communicate with experts in the field, and to continually develop your own knowledge base and scholarly abilities.

You also will be exposed to patients and patients' families from a vast array of cultural, ethnic, religious, socioeconomic, and educational backgrounds including: homeless men, women, and children who live on the streets of major cities; young single mothers; children suffering from asthma; children and adults with HIV/AIDS; academic scholars; and migrant workers, among others. Nursing students—under the guidance of well-qualified faculty—have many opportunities to touch and be touched by the lives of others who may be vastly different from themselves. Such experiences with diverse populations contribute to the students' understanding of human beings, as well as to their ability to provide culturally sensitive care.

Learning to Network

As a student advancing your education, you should plan to take advantage of a wide range of professional opportunities that are available at your college or university, in the local or regional nursing community, and at the national level. For example, lectures given by national and international nursing leaders provide important opportunities to learn about professional, educational, and clinical issues.

Participation in student government, the school's chapter of the National Student Nurses Association (for those studying at the undergraduate level), or the school's chapter of Sigma Theta Tau International, the Honor Society of Nursing, provides an opportunity to develop leadership roles, interact with nursing leaders and scholars, and participate in the political process to influence positive change.

You may want to attend a meeting of the American Nurses Association (ANA), a State Nurses Association (e.g., the New York State Nurses Association), or a meeting of a specialty group (e.g., the American Association of Critical Care Nurses or the Oncology Nursing Society). These meetings will help you learn the newest approaches to caring for patients, families, and communities, and you will also witness how associations work and how nurses influence policy formulation.

Those interested in careers as nurse managers or executives should plan to attend local or national meetings of the American Organization of Nurse Executives (AONE) to appreciate the kind of issues nurses in such positions must address (e.g., staffing, workforce development, fiscal management) and to learn new approaches to dealing with such issues.

Students interested in careers as nurse educators should plan to attend the National League for Nursing (NLN) Educational Summit, where they will have the opportunity to interact with nurse educators from a variety of programs as they explore new approaches to teaching and learning, the research that underlies nursing education, and innovative curriculum and program designs.

All of these types of extracurricular experiences serve to enhance the learning of all students, and you should look for and, indeed, create opportunities to benefit from such experiences. As a student continuing your education, you will be expected to seek out learning opportunities that will help you to meet your professional goals.

Student Responsibility for Learning

Although faculty design programs and courses and engage students in classroom or online discussions, clinical experiences, and assignments (e.g., term papers, community projects, etc.), it is the student who is responsible for his or her own learning. Students often are most successful in nursing education programs when they prepare for class and clinical, ask questions to clarify misunderstandings, and thoughtfully reflect on the ideas or concepts presented. Therefore, you should seek assistance (e.g., from the school's writing center) as needed, meet regularly with faculty advisors, devote uninterrupted time to studying, manage your time well, take advantage of learning opportunities presented to you (e.g., serving on the school's curriculum committee), and seek out learning experiences that will meet your personal needs and goals.

Such assertive behavior may not be comfortable for many students, so you may benefit from talking with your faculty advisor or course instructor about your role in a course. Counseling centers at the school also offer services (e.g., study skills, writing skills, test-taking skills, time management, tutoring, and stress management) that may be of benefit. It is important to seek out and use resources such as these; in fact, they have been created at schools because so many students— both U.S.- and foreign-educated—need such support systems. Each of us has the right and responsibility to secure a quality education that will help us to meet our personal and professional career goals.

STUDENT RIGHTS AND RESPONSIBILITIES

The United States was built on the notion of the supremacy of the rights of human beings. Indeed, the U.S. Declaration of Independence— the founding document of our republic—asserts the right to life, liberty, and the pursuit of happiness. Many states, schools, and programs have developed their own Students' Bill of Rights to outline what students can expect of their education.

Students' Rights

Included among the rights listed in many of these institution-based documents are the following:

- The right to ask questions or express opinions and points of view without being censored or punished.
- The right to be respected as a learner.
- The right to receive timely, helpful, unbiased feedback on one's performance.
- The right to have adequate resources that support successful achievement of outcomes.
- The right to know what is expected of one as a learner.
- The right to be taught by qualified faculty.
- The right to have opportunities to pursue individual interests while enrolled in an academic program.
- The right to know how, when, by whom, and the criteria by which one will be evaluated.
- The right to evaluate one's own progress, strengths, and areas in need of improvement.

Students' Responsibilities

Rights are always accompanied by responsibilities. Among the responsibilities that students are expected to fulfill are the following:

- The responsibility to ask questions or express opinions and points of view that will enhance one's learning and understanding.
- The responsibility to respect faculty and one's fellow students.
- The responsibility to seriously consider and respond to feedback that has been provided regarding one's performance.
- The responsibility to make full use of resources that support successful achievement of outcomes.
- The responsibility to fulfill the expectations of learners that are articulated by faculty.
- The responsibility to provide thoughtful, helpful, unbiased feedback to faculty.
- The responsibility to articulate personal goals and individual interests, and take advantage of or seek out opportunities that will help meet those personal goals and individual interests.
- The responsibility to ask for clarification regarding how, when, by whom, and the criteria on which one will be evaluated, if such information is not provided by faculty.
- The responsibility to evaluate one's own progress, strengths, and areas in need of improvement in a thoughtful way.

SUMMARY

As nursing and nursing education in the United States continue to develop in exciting ways, the opportunities for students are almost unlimited. Students and faculty have much to offer one another and much to learn from one another.

Within a higher education context that is increasingly learner-centered and that emphasizes mutual, collaborative learning, U.S. nursing programs provide incredibly rich environments for students and faculty from all backgrounds to study and learn together. Just as interaction with patients and families of diverse backgrounds enhances the lives of nurses in practice, interaction with fellow students from diverse backgrounds enhances the lives of nursing students and faculty.

This is an exciting time for nursing and nursing education. If you continue to study nursing after you immigrate to the United States, you can expect to be challenged, involved, excited, and supported as you meet your personal and professional goals.

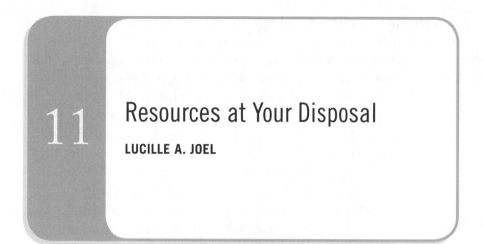

Resources at Your Disposal

LUCILLE A. JOEL

In This Chapter

Keywords

Apprenticeship: Where one works with a skilled professional as a trainee.

Ethnocentrism: The belief in the relative superiority of one's own cultural group.

Curiosity and the capacity to appreciate differences are the greatest resources in adapting to a new country and nursing practice. Each country has the right to sovereignty over the service it expects from its professionals and the manner in which those services are to be offered. This chapter describes some of the resources available that will ease your transition into U.S. culture and help you to understand the profession of nursing as it is practiced in the United States.

The United States can be especially difficult to comprehend, given that we are one from many. We are a people of immigrants, where each group has struggled to maintain its particular national identity. Most immigrants eventually become assimilated into the U.S. culture, while still retaining much of the best of their country of origin.

What are the values of the U.S. population, and how have they changed in recent years? How does U.S. nursing differ from nursing in other parts of the world? What are the inevitable challenges you will find in the United States, and what are the resources at your disposal to make this adventure, be it temporary or permanent, successful?

CONTACT WITH THE COMMUNITY OF THE UNITED STATES

Success is more dependent on great citizens than great leaders (Lamm, 2006), and citizens do not always equate with followers, although when citizens choose to follow, they are unbeatable. Citizens in a great democracy are focused on the future because they believe in something, and they believe that they can make a difference. They feel responsible for the legacy they leave to their children.

The U.S. ethic never has been to let the future take care of itself (Joel, 1998). To Americans, democracy has always required that citizens fully participate in decisions that affect their lives, and excuses to avoid this obligation are unacceptable. This philosophy could just as easily be transferred to the profession of nursing.

Community Involvement

In the best of all worlds, nurses should be involved and invested in three aspects of community life: their profession, their organization or workplace, and their government. Unfortunately, many nurses have not been involved citizens and, additionally, have not treated their outspoken and militant colleagues too kindly. For many among us, it has been easier living with what we know than what we might get with change. Such lack of involvement has been unfortunate in the past. In today's world, it can be downright dangerous.

In recent years, the U.S. population has become more dependent on government for safety and welfare, most especially the state governments. Historically, this has not been the heritage of the United States, a country forged on the tradition of freedom, personal autonomy, and responsibility. We have been a humanitarian and generous people, and it remains highly debatable just how much government in our lives is good. This has been a major issue in every political campaign of memory.

THE PROFESSIONS IN THE UNITED STATES

In 1915, the work of Abraham Flexner, funded by the Carnegie Rockefeller Foundation, set a standard for the professions that has persisted to this day. Flexner proposed six criteria for a profession to be identified as such:

> intellectual, possessing an expanding body of knowledge, unique and socially necessary, taught through a system of professional education as opposed to an **apprenticeship,** internally organized in a manner that allows peer accountability and independence, and motivated through altruism.

These criteria ring just as true today as they did some 95 years ago, but they must be reinterpreted for contemporary use. Later scholars added their own perspectives and enriched our understanding. In total, there is little disagreement. Neither is there any profession, even the most historically recognized, that can claim to be untouched by our changing times. (Joel, 2006, p. 167)

Characteristics of Professions

Although Flexner was the first to speak out on professionalism, many other authors followed him on the topic. Synthesizing the thinking of the best and the brightest, professions hold the following characteristics:

- A profession uses in its practice a well-defined and well-organized body of knowledge that is intellectual in nature and describes its phenomena of concern.
- A profession constantly enlarges the body of knowledge it uses and subsequently imposes on its members the life-long obligation to remain current in order to "do no harm."
- A profession entrusts the education of its practitioners to institutions of higher education.
- A profession applies its body of knowledge in practical services that are vital to human welfare, and especially suited to the tradition of seasoned practitioners shaping the skills of newcomers to the role.
- A profession functions autonomously (with authority) in the formulation of professional policy and in the monitoring of its practice and practitioners.
- A profession is guided by a code of ethics that regulates the relationship between professional and client.
- A profession is distinguished by the presence of a specific culture, norms, and values that are common among its members.
- A profession has a clear standard of educational preparation for entry into practice.
- A profession attracts individuals of intellectual and personal qualities who exalt service above personal gain and who recognize their chosen occupation as a life's work.
- A profession strives to compensate its practitioners by providing freedom of action, opportunity for continuous professional growth, and economic security. (Joel, 2006, pp. 167–168)

Professional Autonomy

By virtue of our Nurse Practice Acts (state laws that govern nursing practice and in some states, nursing education), nursing has been the recipient of professional autonomy as awarded by the public.

Autonomy, as applied to nursing, signifies that no other profession or administrative force can control nursing practice. It also means that the nurse has the freedom to make judgments in patient care within the scope of nursing practice, as defined by the profession and endorsed by the licensing board.

The public expects that the professions will establish standards and monitor the practice of their own members. Professional autonomy is a courtesy given to experts in a complex area of work. Therefore, the nurse has a duty to the employer for the conditions of employment, but a commitment to the patient for the care he or she renders within that role as employee.

LICENSURE: THE GATEWAY TO PRACTICE

In the United States, the state is responsible for the health and welfare of its citizens and, consequently, for the licensing of its health care providers. The state legislature determines which groups are licensed and their specific scopes of practice. In other words, the limits of their practice are identified. Not all health care providers are licensed, but all nurses are in every U.S. state.

It is the responsibility of the executive branch of state government to ensure that law is carried out, including punishment for violations of the law. Given the philosophy of states' rights in the United States, there is the possibility of state-to-state differences, but the licensing laws for nursing in all states and territories include many of the same elements. This is testimony to the strength of nursing organizations that have been vigilant and have looked to maintain conformity.

Nursing Licensure

Individual licensure has meaning beyond ensuring the basic competency of the nurse. The individual license signals the nurse's commitment to the patient, beyond any other, including the employer. The patient's preferences and values are the driving force in the relationship and take precedence over the demands of any employer. This can result in many tense moments in the workplace. You have a responsibility to your employer to respect and follow the conditions of employment and a responsibility to your patients for your practice.

State Boards of Nursing

Each state has a Board of Nursing, which executes the law as contained in the Nurse Practice Act and the administrative code (rules and regulations) that further defines the law. Some states have two boards: one that addresses licensed practical/vocational nursing and one that addresses registered/professional nursing. The majority of states, however, have a single board that oversees both levels of nursing. The state boards come together as peers in the National Council of State Boards of Nursing (NCSBN). The NCSBN offers a robust Web site (http://www.ncsbn.org), which includes links to the individual state boards of nursing and information on licensure in the United States that you may find very useful.

THE ROLE OF THE NURSE IN THE UNITED STATES

The laws governing nursing practice and the requirements of the regulatory agency (Board of Nursing) may seem overwhelming, but with time they should become clear. There are other complex expectations, however, that are essential to nursing in the United States, one of which is cultural competence.

Cultural Competence

Each of us brings the influence of our own cultural heritage, experiences, biases, beliefs, and expectations about patient–nurse relationships to the care that we give. Awareness of the effect of these influences on our caregiving practices is the first step to achieving cultural competence as a nurse. The process of self-assessment must be approached with a willingness to confront and then modify or discard those inaccurate and/or uninformed cultural beliefs and attitudes that detract from the care we provide. Many of our attitudes and beliefs are so ingrained, so deeply a part of us, that we may never examine them in the course of our daily practice until, and if, we become aware of their negative effect on our patients. Even then, long-held biases may limit our introspection.

Ethnocentrism

Ethnocentrism, or the belief in the relative superiority of one's own cultural group, is a common phenomenon. Often operating at an unconscious level, ethnocentrism can exert a powerful influence on our patient interactions and care practices.

If you are unsure whether your approach to a patient is culturally appropriate, acknowledge your unfamiliarity with the patient's cultural norms and ask for guidance in how to best deliver care. Most patients appreciate this consideration and respect and are happy to inform you. Your first rule of practice must be, "Do no harm."

Cultural Communication

How do you assess a patient or community whose primary language is different from your own? What tools or personnel are at your disposal to facilitate assessment, intervention, and teaching? What is your own level of proficiency in English and in languages other than English?

Language competence is essential to quality patient care. With the multicultural patient populations in the United States, many nurses are, or soon will be, challenged in their communication with patients. This becomes a practice issue only if we make no attempt to modify our practice environment to meet the comprehensive needs of our patients. Cultural competency is a required aspect of nursing education in the United States, and in fact, nursing education programs are not accredited without demonstrating this competency.

Autonomy and Assertiveness

In addition to cultural competence, the qualities of assertiveness and autonomy also are essential to nursing practice in the United States. From the patient's perspective, autonomy is the requirement of the health care professional to accept a person's uniqueness, even if the person's values, beliefs, and decisions do not agree with your own. Patients have a right to make the health care decisions that are best suited to their personal philosophies (Joel, 2006). Nurses have the responsibility to truly partner with their patients to provide care that the patient perceives as being respectful and inclusive of his or her uniqueness as a human being. Protection of autonomy is often tricky and may require assertiveness (see chapter 8). It is essential that you know what rights are yours and what rights are your patient's, and be prepared to speak out assertively in defense of both.

THE ROLE OF THE PROFESSIONAL ASSOCIATIONS

The term *semiprofessional* is used widely to signify a field of work that is moving toward the qualities of professionalism detailed earlier, but has not quite arrived. When reviewing the progress of many professions, it is clear that establishing a membership organization to speak for the profession and its professionals is basic and essential. This is particularly important in the United States, where the state awards the individual a license to practice. Professional associations offer a broader world of nursing outside your choice of work environment and provide a source of consultation with a wider perspective.

As you begin a nursing career in the United States, you will find it useful and necessary to join two organizations: a professional nursing organization and one representing your specialty area. The American Nurses Association (ANA) and its state affiliates (e.g., state nurses associations) are considered the professional organizations, where every RN can join and find some way in which to participate. The specialty association (e.g., the Emergency Nurses Association or the Society of Pediatric Nurses) is necessary for you to stay abreast of practice changes in your chosen area of nursing.

The American Nurses Association

The American Nurses Association (ANA) was organized in 1897. It started, and continues, as an organization of nurses, working for nurses.

ANA came into existence for the essential purpose of assuring that the education and practice of nurses was of a sufficient standard to protect the public. Disturbed by the many people with inadequate education who called themselves "nurse," early leaders fought for adequate educational standards for nursing, protection of the title "nurse," and proof of competency in the things that nurses do. In order to give their best to the public, nurses also had the right to demand decent working conditions and safety and security in their work environments. Thus, the economic and general welfare of nurses became a major mission of this newly founded association. These concerns persist today—and addressing them continues to be the major focus of ANA.

ANA Membership

The ANA is a federation of many organizations and individuals. These organizations include state and territorial nurses associations, an association for U.S. nurses overseas, and a federal nurses association composed of members of the U.S. military on active duty. Direct individual membership also is available.

Membership, either through the federation or individually, is exclusive to registered professional nurses; new graduates who are awaiting word of the results of their first experience in taking the U.S. licensing exam, the NCLEX-RN examination; and nurses who have surrendered their licenses as a requirement of a substance abuse treatment program. The varied work of the ANA through its affiliates is presented in Table 11.1.

Knowledge of the work of ANA and the materials it offers is critical as you enter practice in the United States. At the ANA Web site, http://www.nursingworld.org, you will find easy access to position papers on a variety of topics to guide your practice, provide the latest legislative and regulatory news, and more. There also are links to the state nurses associations. See Table 11.2 for a listing of ANA position papers.

The International Council of Nurses

The International Council of Nurses (ICN) is the oldest international association of medical professionals in the world—older than

Table 11.1

SELF-GOVERNING AND INDEPENDENT ORGANIZATIONAL AFFILIATES OF THE AMERICAN NURSES ASSOCIATION (ANA)

NAME	DESCRIPTION OF PURPOSE
The American Academy of Nursing (AAN)	Fellows are elected to membership on the basis of their outstanding contributions to nursing and their potential for continuing contributions, and are entitled to use the initials FAAN after their names.
The American Nurses Foundation (ANF)	A nonmembership organization created for charitable contribution of tax-exempt dollars.
The American Nurses Credentialing Center (ANCC)	A credentialing program established by ANA that awards certification, accreditation, and institutional Magnet status. More than 75,000 advanced practice nurses alone are currently certified by ANCC.
ANA Political Action Committee	A political action group, independent of ANA but related to it. It exists to promote the improvement of health care through education and endorsement of candidates for public office.

the international hospital and medical societies. It is a federation of 128 national nurses associations, representing millions of nurses worldwide. ANA, as the national nurses association of the United States, is the U.S. member of ICN. To become a member, the national association must be autonomous and nondiscriminatory. The membership must be exclusively nurses, and it must reflect the characteristics of nurses in the country and the full range of their concerns, including their education, practice, and economic and general welfare.

These criteria seem simple, but many countries have failed to qualify for membership. ICN works directly with these member associations on the issues of importance to their well-being and global health. The goals of ICN are to bring nurses together worldwide, to advance nurses and nursing worldwide, and to influence health policy.

ICN's Web site, http://www.icn.ch, provides a wide variety of useful information and resources for the migrating nurse. On their Web site, as well as on the CGFNS Web site (http://www.cgfns.org), you

Table 11.2

SAMPLING OF ANA POSITION STATEMENTS

Ethics and Human Rights
- Stem Cell Research
- Use of Placebos for Pain Management in Patients with Cancer
- Reduction of Patient Restraint and Seclusion in Health Care Settings
- Assisted Suicide
- Nurses' Participation in Capital Punishment
- Nursing Care and Do Not Resuscitate Decisions
- Nursing and the Patient Self-Determination Act
- Promotion of Comfort and Relief of Pain in Dying Patients
- The Registered Nurse's Responsibility to Guard Against Working When Fatigued

Bloodborne and Airborne Diseases
- Tuberculosis and HIV
- HIV Exposure from Rape/Sexual Assault
- HIV Disease and Correctional Inmates
- HIV Infection and Nursing Students
- Travel Restrictions for Persons with HIV/AIDS
- HIV/AIDS Disease and Sociocultural Diverse Populations

Social Causes and Health Care
- Physical Violence Against Women
- Eliminating Violence in Advertising Directed Toward Children, Adolescents, and Families
- Childhood Immunizations
- Informal Caregiving
- Discrimination and Racism in Health Care

Drug and Alcohol Abuse
- Position Statement on Opposition to Criminal Prosecution of Women for Use of Drugs While Pregnant
- Drug Testing for Health Care Workers
- Polypharmacy and the Older Adult
- Abuse of Prescription Drugs

Nursing Practice
- Protecting Patient's Safe Access to Therapeutic Marijuana/Cannabis
- Professional Role Competence
- Assuring Safe, High-Quality Care in Pre-K Through 12 Educational Settings

(Continued)

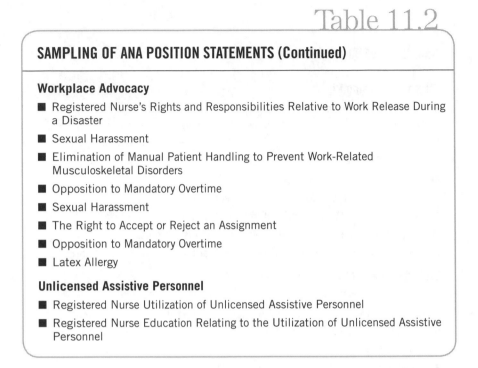

Table 11.2

SAMPLING OF ANA POSITION STATEMENTS (Continued)

Workplace Advocacy

- Registered Nurse's Rights and Responsibilities Relative to Work Release During a Disaster
- Sexual Harassment
- Elimination of Manual Patient Handling to Prevent Work-Related Musculoskeletal Disorders
- Opposition to Mandatory Overtime
- Sexual Harassment
- The Right to Accept or Reject an Assignment
- Opposition to Mandatory Overtime
- Latex Allergy

Unlicensed Assistive Personnel

- Registered Nurse Utilization of Unlicensed Assistive Personnel
- Registered Nurse Education Relating to the Utilization of Unlicensed Assistive Personnel

will find information on the International Centre on Nurse Migration, a joint endeavor between ICN and CGFNS. The Centre plays a key role in establishing global and national migration policy that facilitates safe patient care and positive practice environments for nurse migration. The Centre may be accessed directly at http://www.intlnurse migration.com. You are encouraged to look at all three Web sites.

The Specialty Associations

Once you enter the workforce in the United States, you become specialized. This is inevitable given the scientific and technological complexity of care in the United States. It becomes very difficult to move from one specialty area to another without an investment in education to enable that transition; therefore, it is important to choose wisely as you anticipate your first position.

From another perspective, do not be afraid of cross-training. This is a situation where an employer may request that you train to work in two specialty areas, and it is best if they are related to one another: for example, pediatrics and the new-born nursery, gynecology and the post-partum floor, or gerontology and adult health.

Recognize also that the extent of specialization may be linked to your place of employment. The small community hospital often contains many specialties, and you may be expected to "float," or to move comfortably from one area to another. The need for cross-training definitely applies in this situation. Nurses are responsible for their own practice, and agreeing to work in an area in which you are unprepared can result in serious outcomes for both you and the patient.

Growth of Specialty Associations

There are many specialty organizations and associations in the United States, and the numbers continue to grow. As a field matures, it becomes more specialized, and leaders in these areas of specialization come together for adequate education and practice experiences to ensure competency. This is best done through a specialty association, which provides the peer support needed to accomplish these milestones.

In the United States, it has become tradition that the specialty association works in partnership with ANA to author statements on the scope and standards of practice of the specialty. These standards then become the basis for certification in many specialties. It is important to note that practice in a specialized area and practice as a specialist are two different things. The former comes about from experience and informal and continuing education, and the latter assumes a master's degree in advanced practice with a defined clinical area of study (Joel, 2006). Both are necessary.

The first of the specialty associations was the American Association of Nurse Anesthetists (1931). It was soon followed in the 1940s and 1950s by the American Association of Occupational Health Nurses (formerly the American Association of Industrial Nurses), the Association of Perioperative Nurses (formerly the Association of Operating Room Nurses), and the American College of Nurse Midwives. Beginning in 1968, literally dozens of other specialty associations were organized as the profession became more specialized,

Table 11.3

MAJOR NURSING SPECIALTY ORGANIZATIONS

ORGANIZATION	ESTABLISHED	MEMBERSHIP	ACTIVITIES
Academy of Medical-Surgical Nurses http://amsn.nurse.com	1992	5,000 and 20 local chapters	Standards, publications, research activities
American Association of Neuroscience Nurses http://www.aann.org	1968	3,400 in 60 regional chapters	Certification,[a] standards, legislative and research activities, publications
American Association of Nurse Anesthetists http://www.aana.com	1931	Almost 30,000 (95% CRNAs)	Certification, standards, legislative and research activities, publications
American Association of Occupational Health Nurses http://www.aaohn.org	1942	13,000 with 184 local, state, constituent associations	Certification, standards, legislative and research activities, publications
American Holistic Nurses Association http://www.ahna.org	1980	2,100	Certification, standards, legislative and research activities, publications
American Nephrology Nurses Association http://www.annanurse.org	1969	11,900 in 112 local chapters	Certification, standards, legislative and research activities, publications
American Psychiatric Nurses Association http://www.apna.org		4,500	Certification, standards, legislative and research activities, publications
American Public Health Association, Nursing Section http://www.csuchico.edu/~horst/		1,700	Standards, legislative and research activities, publications
American Society of Plastic Surgical Nurses http://www.aspsn.org	1975	1,700	Certification, standards, research activities, publications
Association for Professionals in Infection Control http://www.apic.org	1972	10,000 multidisciplinary	Certification, standards, legislative and research activities, publications

(Continued)

Table 11.3

MAJOR NURSING SPECIALTY ORGANIZATIONS (Continued)

ORGANIZATION	ESTABLISHED	MEMBERSHIP	ACTIVITIES
Association of Women's Health, Obstetric & Neonatal Nurses http://www.awhonn.org	1969	28,000 in 11 geographic districts	Certification, standards, legislative and research activities, publications
Association of Nurses in AIDS Care http://www.anacnet.org	1987	2,600 in 33 chapters and 3 international affiliates	Certification, standards, legislative and research activities, publications
Association of Perioperative Registered Nurses http://www.aorn.org	1954	41,000 in 340 chapters and 12 specialty assemblies	Certification, standards, legislative and research activities, publications
Association of Rehabilitation Nurses http://www.rehabnurse.org	1974	6,000 in 63 chapters and 10 special interest groups	Certification, standards, legislative and research activities, publications
Emergency Nurses Association http://www.ena.org	1970	23,350 in 20 countries	Certification, standards, legislative and research activities, publications
National Association of Orthopedic Nurses http://www.orthonurse.org	1980	6,700 in 50 chapters	Certification, standards, legislative and research activities, publications
Oncology Nursing Society http://www.ons.org	1975	32,000 in 206 local chapters, 29 national special interest groups, and 100 chapter special interest groups	Certification, standards, legislative and research activities, publications
Society of Pediatric Nurses http://www.pedsnurses.org	1990	2,000	Standards, research activities, publications
Wound, Ostomy and Continence Nurses Society http://www.wocn.org	1968	4,000	Certification, standards, legislative and research activities, publications

[a] Be aware that certification, as it is used in this table, does not mean that the association directly certifies, but rather in most cases this credential is awarded by a free-standing subsidiary.

and nurses saw the need for these support systems to maintain their edge in practice.

Specialty organizations have several things in common. They provide an opportunity for peers to share experiences and challenges related to the field of practice, continuing education, standard setting, and leadership development. Some groups also offer a certification in the specialty. It would be impossible to list all the specialty organizations in nursing today, so a representative list is provided in Table 11.3. You are urged to make contact through their Web sites. A more inclusive list can be found at http://www.nursingworld.org/especiallyforyou/links.

Advocacy Groups

Among the most helpful groups to you will be associations composed of nurse colleagues from your own country. There are many that have come together, such as the National Association of Hispanic Nurses (http://www.thehispanicnurses.org/), the New York Korean Nurses Association (http://www.nykna.org/), the National American Arab Nurses Association (https://n-aana.org/index.asp), the Philippine Nurses Association of America (http://www.philippinenursesaa.org/), the National Association of Indian Nurses of America, and the National Black Nurses Association (http://www.nbna.org/).

Each of these groups has displayed a major commitment to nurses arriving from their home country and feels a responsibility to help you adjust to life and practice in the United States. In many cases, strong personal and professional relationships are built between the nurse who already has been through the adjustment period of living and working in a new country and the nurse who is in the midst of the same challenge. Other advocacy groups may be found through Internet searches.

SUMMARY

Success in immigration is dependent on a basic understanding of the host country and its people. Further, success requires an appreciation that each ethnic and/or national group is sovereign in its beliefs, attitudes, and ethics. You have not traveled this far to change what is not changeable, but to experience those differences. And you are assured plenty of help, be it from advocacy groups of nurses from your home country, specialty associations that share your focus in nursing practice, or your state nurses association as your most faithful support. It is the state nurses association in partnership with ANA and ICN that most fully demonstrates the inclusiveness that is nursing. First and foremost, we are all nurses, and our differences make us more interesting.

REFERENCES

Joel, L. (1998). On citizenship in a great profession. *The American Journal of Nursing,* *98*(4), 7.

Joel, L. (2006). *The nursing experience* (5th ed.). New York: McGraw-Hill.

Lamm, R. (2006, Spring). Great nations need great citizens. *The Social Contract Journal,* *16*(3), 183–186.

Appendix A: Job Interview Materials

In This Appendix

Sample Résumé

Sample Cover Letter

Sample Thank You Letter

SAMPLE RÉSUMÉ

Rhonda P. Jackson
1855 West Patterson Street
Philadelphia, PA 19104
(123) 456-7890
E-mail: rpjackson@yahoo.com

Objective: Seeking an entry-level management position in an acute care hospital where my extensive professional and practical experience will be fully utilized.

Employment History
2004–Present
All Saints Community Hospital, Philadelphia, PA
Staff Nurse

- Implemented patient care for up to 12 patients per section.
- Coordinated patient care with other departments.
- Educated patients/families on health care needs, conditions, options, etc.

- Supervised full- and part-time staff nurses.
- Evaluated staffing requirements, including patient assignments.

Education
2007–2009: Boston College, Boston, MA: MSc in Health Care Management
2000–2004: Philadelphia University, Philadelphia, PA: Bachelor of Science in Nursing

Professional Affiliations
American Nurses Association
Pennsylvania Nurses Association

References
Available upon request

SAMPLE COVER LETTER

Rhonda P. Jackson
1855 West Patterson Street
Philadelphia, PA 19104
(123) 456-7890
rpjackson@yahoo.com
May 2, 2009

Fred Clarkson, MBA
Director of Human Resources
Prince George's Medical Center
323 South Franklin Drive
Baltimore, Maryland 21075

Dear Mr. Clarkson:

Please accept this letter of application for your advertised position of assistant nurse manager in adult health nursing. I have more than five years of nursing experience in adult health and am currently working at All Saints Community Hospital in Philadelphia, PA. During the past 2 years of my nursing career I have obtained a Master's degree in health care management and have taken on increasing management responsibilities on my clinical unit.

I will be relocating to the Baltimore area in July of this year and am interested in moving into a nursing management position in a large, acute care hospital. I look forward to hearing from you regarding an interview at your convenience. You may contact me at: (123) 456-7890 or by E-mail at rpjackson@yahoo.com.

Respectfully,
Rhonda P. Jackson
Enclosure: Résumé

SAMPLE THANK YOU LETTER

Rhonda P. Jackson
1855 West Patterson Street
Philadelphia, PA 19104
(123) 456-7890
May 18, 2009

Fred Clarkson, MBA
Director of Human Resources
Prince George's Medical Center
323 South Franklin Drive
Bladensburg, Maryland 20072

Dear Mr. Clarkson:

Thank you for the opportunity to meet with you and to see your facilities last Wednesday. Both the interview and the tour made for an exciting and complete day. I was particularly impressed with the adult health units of the hospital and the shared governance model that you have instituted. It was very apparent that your staff enjoys working within this model.

Again, thank you for your kindness during my visit and for your efforts in arranging my interview and tour. I look forward to your decision.

Sincerely,
Rhonda P. Jackson

In This Appendix

Immigration and Naturalization Service (INS) 2002 Memo on H-1B Requirements

Citizenship and Immigration Service (CIS) 2005 Memo on Sponsoring Foreign Nurses as Nonimmigrants and Immigrants

Glossary of Selected Visa Terms

Frequently Asked Questions and Answers About Admission Into the United States

IMMIGRATION AND NATURALIZATION SERVICE (INS) 2002 MEMO ON H-1B REQUIREMENTS

U.S. Department of Justice
Immigration and Naturalization Service

HQISD 70/6.2.8-P

Office of the Executive Associate
Commissioner

425 I Street NW
Washington, DC 20536

November 27, 2002

MEMORANDUM FOR REGIONAL DIRECTORS
SERVICE CENTER DIRECTORS
DIRECTOR, ADMINISTRATIVE APPEALS OFFICE
DEPUTY EXECUTIVE ASSOCIATE COMMISSIONER,
IMMIGRATION SERVICES DIVISION

FROM: Johnny N. Williams /S/
Executive Associate Commissioner
Office of Field Operations

SUBJECT: Guidance on Adjudication of H-1B Petitions Filed on
Behalf of Nurses

The purpose of this memorandum is to provide field offices with guidance on adjudication of H-1B petitions when the beneficiary is a registered nurse (RN). This memorandum clarifies that while typical RNs generally do not meet the requirements for H-1B classification, aliens in certain specialized RN occupations are more likely than typical RNs to be eligible for H-1B status.

A. General Requirements for H-1B Classification in a Specialty Occupation

The Service will approve an H-1B nonimmigrant worker petition filed on behalf of certain foreign nurses if the statutory and regulatory requirements for H-1B classification are met. An individual is eligible for H-1B nonimmigrant classification if he or she is in a specialty occupation. Under section 214(i)(1) of the Immigration and Nationality Act (Act), a specialty occupation "means an occupation that requires (A) theoretical and practical application of a body of highly specialized knowledge, and (B) attainment of a bachelor's or higher degree in the specific specialty (or its equivalent) as a minimum for entry into the occupation in the United States." Under section 214(i)(2) of the Act, the specialty occupation requirement is met by "(A) full state licensure to practice in the occupation, if such licensure is required to practice in the occupation, (B) completion of the degree described in paragraph (1)(B) for the occupation, or (C)(i) experience in the specialty equivalent to the completion of such degree, and (ii) recognition of expertise in the specialty through progressively responsible positions relating to the specialty."[1] (C)(i) experience in the specialty equivalent to the completion of such degree, and (ii) recognition of expertise in the specialty through progressively responsible positions relating to the specialty."

An employer may submit evidence that the alien has the required degree (or its equivalent) by submitting:

1. A copy of the alien's U.S. bachelor's or higher degree in the specialty occupation,
2. A copy of the foreign degree determined to be equivalent to the U.S. degree, or
3. Evidence that the alien's education and experience are equivalent to the required U.S. degree.

In order to be licensed as an RN, an individual must graduate from an approved nursing program and pass the National Council Licensure Examination for Registered Nurses (NCLEX-RN) exam. The minimum requirement for entry into the field of nursing as a registered nurse is a two-year associate degree in nursing (AD), meaning a typical RN would not likely be eligible for H-1B classification. (*See* Bureau of Labor Statistics, U.S. Dep't of Labor, *Occupational Outlook Handbook*, 2002–2003 edition, p. 269.) Accordingly, RN positions do not generally require a bachelor's or higher degree. In order to qualify an RN position as H-1B, the petitioning employer can meet the existing regulatory requirements by showing that:

1. A bachelor's or higher degree (or its equivalent) is normally the minimum requirement for entry into the position;
2. The degree requirement is common to the industry for parallel nursing positions (i.e., employers in the same industry require their employees to hold the degree when they are employed in the same or a similar position);

---

[1] An H-1B petition filed for an alien who does not have a valid state license shall be approved for a period of one year provided that the only obstacle to obtaining state license is the fact that the alien cannot obtain a social security card from the Social Security Administration. *See* attached Service memorandum, *Social Security Cards and the Adjudication of H-1B Petitions*, November 20, 2001.

3. The employer normally requires a degree or its equivalent for the position; or

4. The nature of the position's duties is so specialized and complex that the knowledge required to perform the duties is usually associated with the attainment of a bachelor's or higher degree (or its equivalent).

In determining degree equivalencies, the Service uses a formula that requires the beneficiary to have three years of specialized training and/or work experience for each year of college-level training that the beneficiary is lacking. 8 CFR 214.2(h)(4)(iii)(D)(5). The Service will be issuing more detailed technical guidance on this subject in the near future.

Accordingly, a registered nurse will be eligible for H-1B classification if the petitioner can demonstrate that the position and the individual alien meet the requirements for establishing that the position is H-1B as outlined above.

B. Advanced Practice Nurses

In contrast to most general RN positions, certain specialized nursing occupations are likely to require a bachelor's or higher degree, and accordingly, be H-1B equivalent. Positions that require nurses who are certified advanced practice registered nurses (APRN) will generally be H-1B equivalent due to the advanced level of education and training required for certification. An employer may require that the prospective employees hold advanced practice certification as one of the following: clinical nurse specialist (CNS), certified registered nurse anesthetist (CRNA), certified nurse-midwife (CNM), or certified nurse practitioner (APRN-certified). If the APRN position also requires that the employee be certified in that practice, then the nurse will be required to possess an RN, at least a Bachelor of Science in Nursing (BSN), and some additional graduate level education.

The following list describes certain advanced practice occupations that will generally be H-1B equivalent if the position requires, and the alien has obtained, advanced practice certification:

- *Clinical Nurse Specialists (CNS):* Acute Care, Adult, Critical Care, Gerontological, Family, Hospice and Palliative Care, Neonatal, Pediatric, Psychiatric and Mental Health-Adult, Psychiatric and Mental Health-Child, and Women's Health
- *Nurse Practitioner (NP):* Acute Care, Adult, Family, Gerontological, Pediatric, Psychiatric & Mental Health, Neonatal, and Women's Health.
- *Certified Registered Nurse Anesthetist (CRNA);* and
- *Certified Nurse-Midwife (CNM).*

C. Nurses in Administrative Positions

Certain other nursing occupations, such as an upper-level "nurse manager" in a hospital administration position, may be H-1B equivalent since administrative positions typically require, and the individual must hold, a bachelor's degree. (*See* Bureau of Labor Statistics, U.S. Dep't of Labor, *Occupational Outlook Handbook* at 269.) Nursing Services Administrators are generally supervisory level nurses who hold an RN, and a graduate degree in nursing or health administration. (*See* Bureau of Labor Statistics, U.S. Dep't of Labor, *Occupational Outlook Handbook* at 75.)

D. State Requirements

As stated earlier in this memo, a general RN position does not qualify as H-1B. However, the National Council on State Boards of Nurses (NCSBN) has confirmed that the state of North Dakota is the only state that requires that an individual possess a BSN in order to be licensed as an RN in that state. This applies to individuals who enrolled in a nursing program after January 1, 1987. In a situation in which the BSN is a prerequisite to practicing in the field, the position will qualify as an H-1B position. Thus, a petition for an RN position in the state of North Dakota will generally qualify as an H-1B position due to the degree requirement for licensure. The Service will issue updated field guidance if it becomes aware of other states that adopt this requirement.

E. Nursing Specialties

An increasing number of nursing specialties, such as critical care and peri-operative (operating room), to name two examples, require a higher degree of knowledge and skill than a typical RN or staff nurse position. Further, certification examinations are available to registered nurses who are not advanced practice nurses, but who possess additional clinical experience. Examples of these types of certification examinations are school health, occupational health, rehabilitation nursing, emergency room nursing, critical care, operating room, oncology and pediatrics. In such nursing specialties, the petitioner may be able to demonstrate that the H-1B petition is approvable by demonstrating that the position meets the requirements outlined in Section A above, and by demonstrating that the individual nurse meets the requirements. For example, for certain critical care nurses the employer must demonstrate, through affidavits from independent experts or other means, that the nature of the position's duties are sufficiently specialized and complex that the knowledge required to perform the duties is usually associated with the attainment of a bachelor's or higher degree (or its equivalent). As always, each petition must be adjudicated on a case-by-case basis and a decision to approve or deny the petition must take into account the totality of the requirements for the position, (i.e., educational requirements, additional training in the specialty, and the experience), and the individual's qualifications for the position.

Questions regarding this memorandum may be directed to the Office of Adjudications through appropriate channels.

CITIZENSHIP AND IMMIGRATION SERVICE (CIS) 2005 MEMO ON SPONSORING FOREIGN NURSES AS NONIMMIGRANTS AND IMMIGRANTS

Office of Business Liaison

Employer Information Bulletin
19 Guide for Hiring Foreign Nurses

EBISS: (800) 357-2099
NCSC: (800) 375-5283
TDD: (808) 767-1833

November 21, 2005

Fax: (202) 272-1865
Order Forms:
(800) 870-3676
Website:

U.S. Department of Homeland Security:
U.S. Citizenship and Immigration Services

The following is not intended to be legal advice pertaining to your situation and should not be construed as such. The information provided is intended merely as a general overview with regard to the subject matter covered.

Sponsoring Foreign Nurses as Nonimmigrants and Immigrants

Sponsoring Nonimmigrant Foreign Nurses

Nonimmigrant visa options for nurses are limited. Which combination of foreign nursing credentials and U.S. nursing position requirements will qualify for which classification(s) require a fact-based determination. In some cases, more than one alternative may be available. In some cases, no alternative may be available.

H-1A

The H-1A classification for foreign nurses is no longer available. This was a program authorized by Congress in the Nursing Relief Act of 1989 for five years. The program expired on September 1, 1995.

H-1B

The H-1B is not designed specifically for foreign nurses, but for aliens coming to the United States temporarily to provide services in a "specialty occupation" or as a fashion model of distinguished merit and ability.

H-1C[2]

The H-1C classification for foreign nurses is no longer available. The program authorized by Congress through the Nursing Relief for Disadvantaged Area Act of 1999 expired on June 13, 2005. No applications for initial H-1C status or for extension of H-1C status will be accepted. Those who are currently in H-1C status may maintain such status until his or her current visa expires, assuming that the individual continues to satisfy the terms and conditions of H-1C status.

H-2B[3]

The H-2B status affords U.S. employers the ability to bring skilled or unskilled workers from foreign countries to temporarily engage in nonagricultural employment in the United States based on temporary need. Since most U.S. nursing positions constitute permanent employment (this determination is made by the U.S. Department of Labor rather than by the employer), an H-2B petition for a foreign nurse will rarely be approved because the H-2B classification requires that the employer's need to fill the position must be temporary.

TN[4]

Under the North America Free Trade Agreement (NAFTA), a citizen of Canada or Mexico may work in a professional occupation in the United States provided that: (1) the profession is on the NAFTA list, (2) the alien possesses the specific criteria for that profession, (3) the prospective position requires someone in that professional capacity, and (4) the alien is going to work for a U.S. employer. The NAFTA classification, TN, includes 63 professions. The registered nurse is one of the 63 professions. For additional information about admission of Canadian or Mexican nurses as TN aliens under NAFTA, consult Employer Information Bulletin 11.

---

[2] See 20 CFR 655.
[3] See Employer Information Bulletin 8.
[4] See Employer Information Bulletin 11.

H-1B "Specialty Occupation"[5]

Since the expiration of the H-1A category, some petitioning employers have sought to have registered nurses (RNs) classified as eligible for H-1B visas. However, most nurses do not typically meet the requirements for H-1B classification. Nursing, per se, is not a specialty occupation. Whether a particular nursing position qualifies as a specialty occupation depends on the specific facts of that particular case. Aliens in certain specialized RN occupations are more likely than typical RNs to be eligible for H-1B status.

If a prospective employer believes that a particular RN may qualify as an H-1B nonimmigrant, the prospective employer may file a Form I-129 with the appropriate Service Center. RNs do not typically meet the general requirements for H-1B Specialty Occupation Classification.

A specialty occupation is defined as a field of employment, which requires:

(A) Theoretical and practical application of a body of highly specialized knowledge; and

(B) A bachelor's or higher degree in the specific specialty (or its foreign degree equivalent), which is a minimum for entry into the occupation in the United States.

H-1B status generally is not available to most RNs because every state and the District of Columbia permits a person who does not hold a bachelor's degree in nursing, but who meets the educational and testing requirements set by law, to obtain an RN license. Nonetheless, certain nurses may be able to meet statutory and regulatory requirements and receive H-1B approval by establishing that they practice in a specialized field of nursing that does require a bachelor's degree in nursing as the minimum for entry into the specialty.

---

[5] See November 2002 memo, Guidance on Adjudication of H-1B Petitions Filed on Behalf of Nurses 11/27/02 Johnny N. Williams HQOPS (Services/H-1).

NOTE: The fact that a particular RN, in fact, has a Bachelor of Science in Nursing (BSN) is not, by itself, enough to make that RN eligible for H-1B classification. The critical factor is that a person is not *required* to have a BSN in order to obtain a license as an RN. Since one can enter the field of Registered Nursing with something less than a BSN, Registered Nursing is not, itself, a specialty occupation.

Until recently, USCIS recognized an exception for RNs licensed in North Dakota. At one time, North Dakota law provided that no one who enrolled in a nursing program after January 1, 1987 was eligible for licensure as an RN without first obtaining a BSN. Chapter 361 of the 2003 North Dakota Session Laws, however, repealed this requirement. Since this amendment became effective (August 1, 2003), North Dakota now allows a person who has graduated from an approved RN program and who passes the required examination to be licensed as an RN, even if the person does not hold a BSN.

Specialty Occupation Requirements

(A) Full state licensure to practice in the occupation, if such licensure is required to practice in the occupation;[6]

(B) Completion of the degree required for the occupation; or

(C) (i) Experience in the specialty equivalent to the completion of such degree (in other words, have a combination of education, training, and work experience in the specialty occupation equivalent to a U.S. bachelor's degree or higher); and (ii) Recognition of expertise in the specialty through progressively more responsible positions relating to the specialty.

In order to qualify an RN position as an H-1B, the petitioning employer must show:

---

[6] A registered nurse needs to be fully licensed in the state in which they will work. In order to be licensed as an RN, an individual must look to see what the state they will work in requires. Some states require that the individual graduate from an approved nursing program and pass the National Council Licensure Examination for Registered Nurses (NCLEX-RN) exam, some states require passing the commission on Graduates of Foreign Nursing Schools (CGFNS) examination and other states require course-by-course evaluations.

- A bachelor or higher degree or equivalent[7] is normally the standard minimum requirement for entry into the particular specialty occupation;[8]
- The degree required for the subject position must be commonly required for similar positions within the employer's/petitioner's industry. Alternatively, the petitioner must demonstrate that the subject position is so complex or unique that it can be performed only by an individual with the degree or equivalent that is listed as a job requirement;
- The employer must normally require the same degree or its equivalent for the subject position;
- The specific duties of the position must be so specialized and complex that knowledge required for performance of the duties is usually associated with attainment of a bachelor level or higher degree

Aliens in Certain Specialized RN Occupations May be Eligible for H-1B Status

Although general RNs will not typically be eligible for H-1B status, certain specialized nursing occupations are likely to require a bachelor's or higher degree as the minimum requirement for entry into that specialized field and, consequently, have a great chance of satisfying the H-1B requirements. Positions that require nurses who are certified advanced practice registered nurses (APRN) will generally be H-1B equivalent due to the advanced level of training and education required for certification. Furthermore, employers may require that the prospective employee hold advanced practice certification (i.e., clinical nurse specialist, certified registered nurse anesthetist, certified nurse-midwife, or certified nurse practitioner). If the APRN

---

[7] A combination of education, training, and work experience may substitute for a bachelor's degree. In such cases, three years of specialized training and/or experience can substitute for one year of college study, if accepted by USCIS.

[8] The reporting of a U.S. or foreign degree is not required in a standard format on any of the USCIS or DOL forms, but is generally provided by the petitioning employer in supporting documentation. In cases where the degree was earned outside of the United States, the employer may have to provide a credentials evaluation stating that the foreign degree is "equivalent to" a particular U.S. degree. USCIS does not certify or recommend credentialing services.

position requires that the employee be certified in that practice, then the nurse will be required to possess an RN, at least a BSN, and some additional graduate level education (such as a master's degree).

It is also important to note that there are also nursing specialties that require a higher degree of knowledge and skill than a typical RN. Certification examinations may be available to RNs who are not advanced practice nurses, but who possess additional clinical experience in certain areas (e.g., school health, occupational health, rehabilitation nursing, emergency room nursing, critical care, operating room, oncology, and pediatrics). The petitioner may be able to demonstrate that the H-1B petition may be approved by demonstrating that the position meets the requirements outlined above and by demonstrating that the individual meets those requirements.

- **Nurses in Administrative Positions**
  Certain other nursing occupations, such as an upper-level "nurse manager" in a hospital administrative position, may be H-1B equivalent since administrative positions typically require, and the individual must hold, a bachelor's degree. (*See* Bureau of Labor Statistics, USDOL, *Occupational Outlook Handbook* at 269.) Nursing Services Administrators are generally supervisory level nurses who hold an RN and a graduate degree in nursing or health administration. (*See* Bureau of Labor Statistics, USDOL, *Occupational Handbook* at 75.)

Sponsoring Foreign Nurses As Lawful Permanent Residents

Issuance of Employment-Based immigrant visas typically involves three main steps. First, the employer must establish, through the labor certification process, that there is a shortage of sufficient workers willing and able to provide the services the alien nurse is to provide and that the immigration of the alien nurse will not adversely affect wage and working conditions in the United States. Second, the Form I-140 is filed at the USCIS Service Center with geographic jurisdiction over the place of employment. Once the Form I-140 is approved and it has been determined that the alien has the minimum requirements, the alien beneficiary becomes eligible to apply for an immigrant visa, once the priority date is current.

If the alien is present in the United States in a lawful status, approval of the Form I-140 may permit the alien to apply for adjustment of status, instead of going abroad to obtain an immigrant visa.

Schedule A: Labor Certification

As noted above, aliens who seek to enter the United States in specified Employment-Based permanent visa categories are excluded from the United States unless the Secretary of Labor has certified to the Secretary of State and Attorney General that there are not sufficient workers who are able, willing, and qualified U.S. workers, and available at the time of application for a visa and admission to the United States and at the place where the alien is to perform such skilled or unskilled labor, and the employment of such alien will not adversely affect the wages and working conditions of U.S. workers similarly employed. This process is normally called a labor certification.

Every petition must be accompanied by an individual labor certification from the DOL or by an application for Schedule A designation. To apply for Schedule A designation, a fully executed uncertified Form ETA 750 in duplicate must accompany the Form I-140 petition.[9]

Schedule A is a list of occupations which have been pre-certified by the DOL and it has been determined that there are not sufficient U.S. workers who are able, willing, qualified, and available for the occupations, and that the wages and working conditions of U.S. workers similarly employed will not be affected by the employment of aliens in Schedule A occupations. Nursing is an occupation that has been pre-certified by the DOL.

It is important to note that this pre-certification only applies to "professional nurses." Professional nurses' duties generally include the making of clinical judgments concerning the observation, care,

---

[9] An employer seeking a Schedule A labor certification as a professional nurse, shall file as part of its labor certification application, documentation that the alien has passed the Commission on Graduates of Foreign Nursing Schools (CGFNS) examination; or that the alien holds a full and unrestricted (permanent) license to practice professional nursing in the state of intended employment.

and counsel of persons requiring nursing care and administering of medicines and treatments prescribed by the physician or dentist; and the participation in activities for the promotion of health and the prevention of illness in others. A program of study for professional nurses generally includes theory and practice in clinical areas such as obstetrics, surgery, pediatrics, psychiatry, and medicine. Certified nurses assistants, licensed vocational nurses, practical nurses, and nurse aids are not professional nurses.

Form I-140

Classification for a nurse will typically be in the third Employment-Based category (EB-3), either skilled worker or professional. Note that, as with the H-1B, a registered nurse would have to work in a position that *requires* a bachelor's degree in order for the registered nurse to qualify for EB-3 classification as a professional. Supporting documentation must be submitted with the Form I-140.

The sponsoring employer should include the following documentation:

- Properly filed petition/Form I-140.
- Either DOL certified labor certification, ETA 750 Parts A and B, or an application for Schedule A designation (uncertified ETA 750 Parts A and B) in duplicate.[10]
- Form G-28 if represented by an attorney.
- Any document containing foreign language submitted to USCIS shall be accompanied by a full English language translation, which the translator has certified as complete and accurate,

---

[10] Professional nurses seeking permanent labor certification on Schedule A must document that he or she passed "the Commission on Graduates of Foreign Nursing Schools (CGFNS) Examination; or...hold a full and unrestricted license to practice professional nursing in the State of intended employment." 20 CFR 656.10. On December 20, 2002, the Immigration and Naturalization Service issued a memorandum addressing the adjudication of the Form I-140 petitions filed on behalf of Schedule A nurses, which was issued pursuant to DOL guidance. Specifically, employers may receive a Schedule A labor certification on behalf of a nurse, if the nurse has successfully passed the National Council Licensure Examination for Registered Nurses (NCLEX-RN) examination in lieu of either having passed the CGFNS examination or being in full possession of a full and unrestricted license to practice nursing in the state of intended employment.

and by the translator's certification that he or she is competent to translate from the foreign language into English.

- Evidence that the prospective U.S. employer has the ability to pay the proffered wage. Evidence of this ability shall be either in the form of copies of annual reports, federal tax returns, or audited financial statements. In appropriate cases, additional evidence, such as profit/loss statements, bank account records, or personnel records may be requested.
- Evidence of the beneficiary's qualifications, such as proof of nursing diploma or degree, proof of nursing registration/licensure from the country where the degree was obtained, etc.[11]

Section 343 of IIRIRA/CGFNS Certification Program

Section 343 of the Illegal Immigration Reform and Immigrant Responsibility Act (IIRIRA), created a new ground of inadmissibility for any immigrant or nonimmigrant alien who seeks to enter the United States to perform labor as a healthcare worker. This rule applies to aliens coming to the United States—whether as immigrants or nonimmigrants for the primary purpose of performing labor in the nursing occupation. Section 343 requires certification that verifies that the nurse's education, training, licensing, experience and English competency. The Commission on Graduates of Foreign Nursing Schools (CGFNS) has been designated to provide the certificate to applicants who seek to perform labor as a professional nurse. As of the date of this Employer Information Bulletin, no other organization has been authorized to provide these certifications for nurses.

---

[11] On October 2, 2002, DOL advised the Immigration and Naturalization Service that, in adjudicating EB-3 petitions on behalf of nurses, the Service may accept documentation that the alien beneficiary has passed the NCLEX-RN examination as eligibility for a Schedule A labor certification in addition to a CGFNS certificate or nurse license. See INS Memorandum December 20, 2002 which instructs all Service Centers to favorably consider the Form I-140 petition for a foreign nurse, as being eligible for a Schedule A labor certification, upon presentation of a certified copy of a letter from the state of intended employment which confirms that the alien has passed the NCLEX-RN examination and is eligible to be issued a license to practice nursing in that state.

Once the screening is successful, the certifying organization (currently, only CGFNS for nurses) issues what is called a Visa Screen certificate. The certificate is evidence that the alien has met the requirements of section 343 of IIRIRA and nothing more. Do not confuse the certificate with other requirements, such as state license requirements and other requirements. The alien must still meet all other regulatory and statutory requirements for the Employment-Based classification sought as well as for adjustment of status. In particular, the issuance of a Visa Screen certificate would not preclude a nurse being sanctioned for practicing in a particular state without any license that that state may require.

Immigrant Visa Processing/Adjustment of Status

A Visa Screen certificate must be obtained before an immigrant visa will be issued. So once the Form I-140 has been approved and a Visa Screen certificate obtained, a nurse is then eligible to apply for an immigrant visa through consular processing. If they are in the United States in a lawful status they may apply to adjust their status to that of a lawful permanent resident.

Contrary to the regulations that once applied to applicants for H-1A visas, there is no requirement that the applicant be certified by the state licensing agency where he or she intends to work. Rather, presentation of the Visa Screen certificate indicates that the alien's education, training, license, and experience suggest that he or she should not have any problem in getting licensed following entry.

For applicants as yet unlicensed in the state in which they intend to work, rather than requiring proof that the alien has enrolled for such testing, the post should just judge the alien's intent to work for the petitioning health care provider. If the post is satisfied that the alien intends to work for the petitioner, it should accept the presumption that the alien will take all necessary steps to follow through on state licensing.

Once in the United States, nurses are required to adhere to licensing requirements of the state in which they intend to work. Requirements vary from state to state. It is imperative to look up each state's requirements.

Nonimmigrants

As noted, section 343 applies to nonimmigrants as well as to immigrants. While working to develop the Visa Screen rules, however, Legacy INS and the Department of State jointly exercised their discretion to waive the foreign health care worker certification requirement for nonimmigrant health care workers.

With the promulgation of the Final Rule on July 25, 2003, the requirements of section 343 now affect the admission of nonimmigrants as well as immigrants. The Final Rule became effective on September 23, 2003, and requires nonimmigrant health care workers to obtain and present certification to the DHS each time they apply for admission, an extension of stay, or a change of status. To provide for a smooth transition, however, the Department of Homeland Security and the Department of State continued to waive the ground of inadmissibility for nonimmigrants seeking admission before July 26, 2004. Until July 26 2004, DHS admitted and approved applications for extensions of stay and/or change of status for nonimmigrant health care workers who had not yet satisfied the Visa Screen requirements. The waiver allowed these aliens temporary admission for a period no longer than one year from the date of the decision. The alien had to obtain the certification within one year of date of admission or decision. This waiver provision expired on July 26, 2004.

Accordingly, on or after July 26, 2004, if an alien seeks admission, change of status, or extension of stay, the alien must provide evidence of the health care worker certification if his or her primary purpose for coming to or remaining in the United States is employment in one of the affected health care occupations.

Aliens who seek admission as TN nonimmigrants under NAFTA are subject to the section 343 certification requirements to the same extent as all other nonimmigrants. On July 22, 2004, however, the Secretary of Homeland Security published an interim regulation, 69 *Fed. Reg.* 43729, amending the Department of Homeland Security regulations to extend until July 26, 2005 the deadline by which certain health care workers from Canada and Mexico must obtain health care worker certifications.

This rule applies only to Canadian and Mexican health care workers who, before September 23, 2003, were employed as "trade NAFTA" (TN) or "trade Canada" (TC) nonimmigrant health care workers and held valid licenses from a U.S. jurisdiction.

A TN nonimmigrant may establish eligibility for the waiver of the health care certification requirement by providing evidence that the initial admission as a TN or TC nonimmigrant health care worker occurred before September 23, 2003, and employment and licensing as a health care worker was before September 23, 2003. Evidence may include, but is not limited to, copies of prior TN or TC approval notices, Forms I-94, employment verification letters, pay stubs, and state health care worker licenses. In addition, DHS electronic records evidencing admission as a TN or TC may be considered.

DHS understands that many TN nonimmigrants actually live in Canada or Mexico and regularly travel to their jobs in the United States. Because many of the aliens protected by this interim rule are regular travelers, it is not necessary for them to have been physically present in the United States on September 23, 2003, in order to benefit from this deadline extension.

This extension does not apply to any alien whose initial admission as a TN nonimmigrant health care worker occurred on or after September 23, 2003. Any alien whose initial admission was on or after September 23, 2003, was admitted on notice of the certification requirement and does not benefit from the additional extension.

An alien whose initial TN admission was on or after September 23, 2003, and before midnight on July 26, 2004, must have the appropriate health care worker certification to be admissible after July 26, 2004, even if applying for admission during a period of time previously authorized on Form I-94 issued at the time of a prior admission between September 23, 2003 and before midnight on July 26, 2004.

Any alien not described in the interim rule who seeks admission after July 26, 2004 to work in a covered health care field will be inadmissible if the alien has not obtained the required certificate. As provided in section 212(d)(3) of the Immigration and Nationality Act and Title 8, Code of Federal Regulations 212.15(n), the Secretary may waive this ground of admissibility on a case-by-case basis.

How Long Will This Process Take?

It is difficult to estimate how long the entire process will take. First, it cannot be estimated how long it takes a foreign nurse to receive his or her CGFNS Certificate. Second, there are different processing times for the Form I-129 or Form I-140 at each USCIS Service Center. In addition, it cannot be estimated how long it will take a foreign nurse to gather the information required to receive his or her Visa Screen certificate as well as be approved for the certificate. Finally, once the approved petition is sent to the U.S. Embassy or Consulate abroad where the nurse applies for the immigrant or nonimmigrant visa, the processing time varies from country to country.

GLOSSARY OF SELECTED VISA TERMS

Accompanying: A type of visa in which family members travel with the principal applicant (in immigrant visa cases, within six months of issuance of an immigrant visa to the principal applicant).

Adjust Status: (1) To change from a nonimmigrant visa status or other status, (2) To adjust the status of a permanent resident (green card holder).

Admission: Entry into the United States is authorized by a Department of Homeland Security, Customs and Border Protection (CBP) officer. When you come from abroad and first arrive in the United States, the visa allows you to travel to the port-of-entry and request permission to enter the United States. Admission or entering the United States, by non-U.S. citizens must be authorized by a CBP officer at the port-of-entry, who determines whether you can enter and how long you can stay here, on any particular visit. If you are allowed to enter, how long you can stay and the immigration classification you are given is shown as a recorded date or Duration of Status (D/S) on Form I-94, Arrival Departure Record, or Form I-94W, if arriving on the Visa Waiver Program. If you want to stay longer than the date authorized, you must request permission from the Department of Homeland Security, U.S. Citizenship and Immigration Services (USCIS).

Advance Parole: Permission to return to the United States after travel abroad granted by DHS prior to leaving the United States. The following categories of people may need advance parole: people on a K-1 visa, asylum applicants, parolees, people with Temporary Protected Status (TPS) and some people trying to adjust status, while in the United States. If these categories of people do not apply for advance parole before they leave the United States, they may be unable to return.

An alien in the United States and applying for an Advance Parole document for him- or herself must attach: (1) a copy of any document issued to the alien by USCIS or former INS showing present status in the United States; and (2) an explanation or other evidence demonstrating the circumstances that warrant issuance of Advance Parole.

If the alien is basing his or her eligibility for Advance Parole on a separate application for adjustment of status or asylum, he must also attach a copy of the filing receipt for that application. If the alien is traveling to Canada to apply for an immigrant visa, he or she must also attach a copy of the consular appointment.

Agent: In immigrant visa processing the applicant selects a person who receives all correspondence regarding the case and pays the immigrant visa application processing fee. The agent can be the applicant, the petitioner, or another person selected by the applicant.

Alien: A foreign national who is not a U.S. citizen.

Applicant (Visa): A foreign citizen who is applying for a nonimmigrant or immigrant U.S. visa. The visa applicant may also be referred as a beneficiary for petition-based visas.

Appointment package: The letter and documents that tell an applicant of the date of the immigrant visa interview. It includes forms that the applicant must complete before the interview and instructions for how to get everything ready for the interview.

Approval notice: A Department of Homeland Security, U.S. Citizenship and Immigration Services (USCIS) immigration form, Notice of Action, Form I-797 that says that USCIS has approved a petition, or request for extension of stay or change of status.

Asylee: An alien in the United States or at a port of entry who is found to be unable or unwilling to return to his or her country of nationality, or to seek the protection of that country because of persecution or a well-founded fear of persecution. Persecution or the fear thereof must be based on the alien's race, religion, nationality, membership in a particular social group, or political opinion. For persons with no nationality, the country of nationality is considered to be the country in which the alien last habitually resided. Asylees are eligible to adjust to lawful permanent resident status after one year of continuous presence in the United States. These immigrants are limited to 10,000 adjustments per fiscal year.

Arrival-departure card: Also known as Form I-94, Arrival-Departure Record. The Department of Homeland Security, Customs and Border Protection official at the port-of-entry gives foreign visitors (all non-U.S. citizens) an Arrival-Departure Record, (a small white card) when they enter the United States. Recorded on this card is the immigrant classification and the authorized period of stay in the United States. This is either recorded as a date or the entry of D/S, meaning duration of status. It is important to keep this card safe because it shows the length of time you are permitted and authorized by the Department of Homeland Security to stay in the United States. It is best kept stapled with your passport, kept in a safe place. The visitors return the I-94 card when they leave the country. The I-94W, Nonimmigrant Visa Waiver Arrival-Departure Record (green card) is for travelers on the Visa Waiver Program.

Biometrics: A biometric or biometric identifier is an objective measurement of a physical characteristic of an individual which, when captured in a database, can be used to verify the identity or check against other entries in the database. The best known biometric is the fingerprint, but others include facial recognition and iris scans.

Case number: The National Visa Center (NVC) gives each immigrant petition a case number. This number has three letters followed by ten digits (numbers). The three letters are an abbreviation for the overseas embassy or consulate that will process the immigrant visa case (for example, GUZ for Guangzhou, CDJ for Ciudad Juarez).

Certificate of Naturalization: A document issued by the Department of Homeland Security as proof that the person has become a U.S. citizen (naturalized) after immigration to the United States.

Child: Unmarried child under the age of 21 years. A child may be natural born, step, or adopted. If the child is a stepchild, the marriage between the parent and the American citizen must have occurred when the child was under the age of 18. If the child is adopted, he/she must have been adopted with a full and final adoption when the child was under the age of 16, and the child must have lived with and been in the legal custody of the parent for at least two years. An orphan may qualify as a child if he/she has been adopted abroad by an American citizen or if the American citizen parent has filed an immediate-relative (IR) visa petition for him/her to go to the United States for adoption by the American citizen.

In certain visa cases a child continues to be classified as a child after he/she becomes 21, if the petition was filed for him/her when he/she was still under 21 years of age. For example, an IR-2 child of an American citizen remains a child after the age of 21 if a petition was filed for him/her on or after August 6, 2002, when he/she was still under 21 years old. The child must meet other requirements of a child as listed above.

Common-law marriage: An agreement between a man and woman to enter into marriage without a civil or religious ceremony. It may not be recognized as a marriage for immigration purposes.

Conditional residence visa: If you have been married for less than two years when your husband or wife (spouse) gets lawful permanent resident status (gets a green card), then your spouse gets residence on a conditional basis. After two years you and your spouse must apply together to the Department of Homeland Security to remove the condition to the residence.

The investor visa (EB5 or T5/C5) is also a conditional residence. It requires an application procedure after two years to remove the condition on the permanent residence.

Current/noncurrent: There are numerical limits on the number of immigrant visas that can be granted to aliens from any one foreign country. The limit is based on place of birth, not citizenship. Because of the numerical limits, this means there is a waiting time before the immigrant visa can be granted. The terms current/noncurrent refer to the priority date of a petition in preference immigrant visa cases in relationship to the immigrant cut-off date. If your priority date is before the cut-off date according to the monthly Visa Bulletin, your case is current. This means your immigrant visa case can now be processed. However, if your priority date is later/comes after the cut-off date, you will need to wait longer, until your priority date is reached (becomes current).

Cut-off date: The date that determines whether a preference immigrant visa applicant can be scheduled for an immigrant visa interview in any given month. The cut-off date is the priority date of the first applicant who could not get a visa interview for a given month. Applicants with a priority date earlier than the cut-off date can be scheduled. However, if your priority date is on or later than the cut-off date, you will need to wait longer, until your priority date is reached (becomes current).

Duration of status: In certain visa categories such as diplomats, students and exchange visitors, the alien may be admitted into the United States for as long as the person is still doing the activity for which the visa was issued, rather than being admitted until a specific departure dates. This is called admission for "duration of status." For students, the time during which a student is in a full course of study plus any authorized practical training, and following that, authorized time to depart the country, is duration of status. The length of time depends upon the course of study. For an undergraduate degree this is commonly four years (eight semesters). Normally the immigration officer gives a student permission to stay in the United States for "duration of status." Duration of Status (or D/S) is recorded on Form I-94, Arrival-Departure Record. The Department of Homeland Security U.S immigration inspector at port-of-entry gives foreign visitors (all non-U.S citizens) an Arrival-Departure Record, (a small white card) when they enter the United States. Recorded on this card is the visa classification and the authorized period of stay in the United States. This is either recorded as a date or the entry or D/S, meaning duration of status. The I-94 is a very important card to make sure you keep, because it shows the length of time you are permitted and authorized by the Department of Homeland Security to stay in the United States.

Department of Labor: The Department of Labor fosters and promotes the welfare of the job seekers, wage earners, and retirees of the United States by improving their working conditions, advancing their opportunities for profitable employment, protecting their retirement and health care benefits, helping employers find workers, strengthening free collective bargaining, and tracking changes in employment, prices, and other national economic measurements. In carrying out this mission, the Department administers a variety of Federal labor laws including those that guarantee workers' rights to safe and healthful working conditions; a minimum hourly wage and overtime pay; freedom from employment discrimination; unemployment insurance; and other income support.

Green card: A wallet-sized card showing that the person is a lawful permanent resident (immigrant) in the United States. It is also known as a permanent resident card (PRC), an alien registration receipt card and I-551. It was formerly green in color.

I-551 (green card): Permanent residence card or alien registration receipt card or "green card." *See* Lawful Permanent Resident.

Immigrant visa: A visa for a person who plans to live indefinitely and permanently in the United States.

Immigration and Nationality Act (INA): The Immigration and Nationality Act, or INA, was created in 1952. Before the INA, a variety of statutes governed immigration law but were not organized in one location. The McCarran-Walter bill of 1952, Public Law No. 82-414, collected and codified many existing provisions and reorganized the structure of immigration law. The Act has been amended many times over the years, but is still the basic body of immigration law.

The INA is divided into titles, chapters, and sections. Although it stands alone as a body of law, the Act is also contained in the United States Code (U.S.C.). The code is a collection of all the laws of the United States. It is arranged in fifty subject titles by general alphabetic order. Title 8 of the U.S. Code is but one of the fifty titles and deals with "Aliens and Nationality." When browsing the INA or other statutes you will often see reference to the U.S. Code citation. For example, Section 208 of the INA deals with asylum, and is also contained in 8 U.S.C. 1158. Although it is correct to refer to a specific section by either its INA citation or its U.S. code, the INA citation is more commonly used.

In status: It's important to understand the concept of immigration status and the consequences of violating that status. Being aware of the requirements and possible consequences will make it more likely that you can avoid problems with maintaining your status. Every visa is issued for a particular purpose and for a specific class of visitor. Each visa classification has a set of requirements that the visa holder must follow and maintain. Those who follow the requirements maintain their status and ensure their ability to remain in the United States. Those who do not follow the requirements violate their status and are considered "out of status." For more information see "Out of Status" below. In Status means you are in compliance with the requirements of your visa type under immigration law. For example, you are a foreign student who entered the United States on a student visa. If you are a full-time student and pursuing your course of study, and are not engaged in unauthorized employment, you are "in status." If you work full time in your uncle's convenience store and do not study, you are "out of status."

Labor Condition Application (LCA): A request to the Department of Labor for a foreign citizen to work in the United States.

Lawful Permanent Resident (LPR): A person who has immigrated legally but is not an American citizen. This person has been admitted to the United States as an immigrant and has a Permanent Resident Card, Form I-551 also known as *green card.* It is a wallet-sized card showing that the person is a lawful permanent resident (immigrant) in the United States. This person is also called a legal permanent resident, a green card holder, a permanent resident alien, a legal permanent resident alien (LPRA) and resident alien permit holder.

Lose status: To stay in the United States longer than the period of time which Department of Homeland Security (DHS) gave to a person when he/she entered the United States, or to fail to meet the requirements or violate the terms of the visa classification. The person becomes "out of status."

Machine Readable Passport (MRP): A passport that has biographic information entered on the data page according to international specifications. A machine readable passport is required to travel with a visa on the Visa Waiver Program.

Machine Readable Visa (MRV): A visa that contains biometric information about the passport holder. A visa that immigration officers read with special machines when the applicants enter the United States. It gives biographic information about the passport holder and tells the Department of Homeland Security (DHS) information on the type of visa. It is also called MRV.

National Visa Center (NVC): A Department of State facility located in Portsmouth, New Hampshire. It supports the worldwide operations of the Bureau of Consular Affairs Visa Office. The NVC processes immigrant visa petitions from the Department of Homeland Security (DHS) for people who will apply for their immigrant visas at embassies and consulates abroad. It also collects fees associated with immigrant visa processing.

Nonimmigrant Visa (NIV): A U.S. visa allows the bearer, a foreign citizen, to apply to enter the United States temporarily for a specific purpose. Nonimmigrant visas are primarily classified according to the principal purpose of travel. With few exceptions, while in the United States, nonimmigrants are restricted to the activity or reason for which their visa was issued. Examples of persons who may receive nonimmigrant visas are tourists, student, diplomats, and temporary workers.

Out of status: A U.S. visa allows the bearer to apply for entry to the United States in a certain classification, for a specific purpose. For example, student (F), visitor (B), temporary worker (H). Every visa is issued for a particular purpose and for a specific class of visitor. Each visa classification has a set of requirements that the visa holder must follow and maintain. When you arrive in the United States, a Department of Homeland Security (DHS) Customs and Border Protection (CBP) inspector determines whether you will be admitted, length of stay and conditions of stay in, the United States. When admitted you are given a Form I-94 (Arrival/Departure Record), which tells you when you must leave the United States. The date granted on the I-94 card at the airport governs how long you may stay in the United States. If you do not follow the requirements, you stay longer than that date, or you engage in activities not permitted for your particular type of visa, you violate your status and are considered to be "out of status." It is important to understand the concept of immigration status and the consequences of violating that status. Failure to maintain status can result in arrest, and violators may be required to leave the United States. Violation of status also can affect the prospect of readmission to the United States for a period of time, by making you ineligible for a visa. Most people who violate the terms of their status are barred from lawfully returning to the United States for years.

Port of entry: Place (often an airport) where a person requests admission to the United States by the Department of Homeland Security, Customs and Border Protection officer.

Priority date: The priority date decides a person's turn to apply for an immigrant visa. In family immigration the priority date is the date when the petition was filed at a Department of Homeland Security (DHS), U.S. Citizenship and Immigration Services office or submitted to an Embassy or Consulate abroad. In employment immigration the priority date may be the date the labor certification application was received by the Department of Labor (DOL).

Sponsor: (1) A person who fills out and submits an immigration visa petition. Another name for sponsor is petitioner, *or* (2) a person who completes an affidavit of support (I-864) for an immigrant visa applicant.

Spouse: Legally married husband or wife. A cohabiting partner does not qualify as a spouse for immigration purposes. A common-law husband or wife may or may not qualify as a spouse for immigration purposes, depending on the laws of the country where the relationship occurs.

Temporary worker: A foreign worker who will work in the United States for a limited period of time. Some visas classes for temporary workers are H,

L, O, P, Q, and R. If you are seeking to come to the United States for employment as a temporary worker (H, L, O, P, and Q visas), your prospective employer must file a petition with the Department of Homeland Security (DHS), USCIS. This petition must be approved by USCIS before you can apply for a visa.

Visa Waiver Program (VWP): The Visa Waiver Program (VWP) enables nationals of certain countries to travel to the United States for tourism or business [visitor (B) visa purposes] for stays of 90 days or less without obtaining a visa. The program was established in 1986 with the objective of eliminating unnecessary barriers to travel, stimulating the tourism industry, and permitting the Department of State to focus consular resources in other areas. VWP eligible travelers may apply for a visa, if they prefer to do so. Not all countries participate in the VWP, and not all travelers from VWP countries are eligible to use the program. VWP travelers are required to apply for authorization though the Electronic System for Travel Authorization (ESTA), are screened at their port of entry into the United States, and are enrolled in the Department of Homeland Security's US visit program.

Glossary of Selected Visa Terms From:
http://www.travel.state.gov/visa/frvi/glossary
http://www.cbp.gov/xp/cgov/travel
http://www.uscis.gov/portal/site/uscis

FREQUENTLY ASKED QUESTIONS AND ANSWERS ABOUT ADMISSION INTO THE UNITED STATES

Q: *What is the Inspection Process?*

A: All persons arriving at a port-of-entry to the United States are subject to inspection by U.S. Customs and Border Protection (CBP) Officers. CBP Officers will conduct the Immigration, Customs, and Agriculture components of the Inspections process. If a traveler has health concerns, he/she will be referred to a Public Health Officer for a separate screening.

Q: *What Does the Law Say?*

A: The legal foundation that requires the inspection of all persons arriving in the United States comes from the Immigration and Nationality Act (INA), see INA § 235 [8 U.S.C.]. Rules published in the Federal Register explain the inspection requirements and process. These rules are incorporated into the Code of Federal Regulations [CFR] at 8 CFR § 235.

Q: *What Can I Expect to Happen at a Port-of-Entry?*

A: **Airport** When arriving at an airport, the airline will give all non-U.S. citizens a form to complete while still en route to the United States, either Form I-94 (white), Arrival/Departure Record, or Form I-94W (green), Nonimmigrant Visa Waiver Arrival/Departure Form and Customs Declaration form 6059B. The forms ask for basic identification information and the address where you will stay in the United States.

Upon arrival, the airline personnel will show you to the inspection area. You will queue up in an inspection line and then speak with a CBP officer. If you are a U.S. citizen, special lines may be available to you. If you are not a U.S. citizen, you should use the lanes marked for non-citizens. If you are a U.S. citizen, the officer will ask you for your passport and Customs Declaration form, verify your citizenship, and welcome you back to the United States. You may be asked to proceed to a second screening point with your belongings for additional questioning by CBP Officers. You will then proceed to the Customs inspection area.

If you are an alien, the CBP Officer must determine why you are coming to the United States, what documents you may require, if you have those documents, and how long you should be allowed to initially stay in the United States. These determinations usually take less than one minute to make. If you are allowed to proceed, the officer will stamp your passport and customs declaration form and issue a completed Form I-94 to you. A completed form I-94 will show what immigration classification you were given and how long you are allowed to stay.

Also, if you are an alien, CBP Officers may decide that you should not be permitted to enter the United States. There are many reasons why this might happen (see INA § 212(a)). You will either be placed in detention, or temporarily held until return flight arrangements can be made. If you have a visa, it may be cancelled. In certain instances, Officer(s) may not be able to decide if you should be allowed into the United States. In this case, your inspection may be deferred (postponed), and you will be instructed to go to another office located near your intended destination in the United States for further processing.

Land At a land border port-of-entry you will undergo the same general process. One officer will conduct the primary inspection on the vehicle lane. That officer may send you for further review or issuance of needed papers to a secondary inspection area. Once a determination is made to allow you into the United States, you may be sent for further Customs inspection or immediately allowed to proceed on your trip. Alien truck drivers may qualify for admission as B-1 visitors for business to pick up or deliver cargo traveling in the stream of international commerce. Please see "How Do I Enter the United States as a Commercial Truck Driver" for more information.

Sea The inspection process at a sea port-of-entry is similar to the airport process if inspection facilities are available. Otherwise passengers will be instructed where to report for inspection on board the vessel.

Q: *What Documents Must I Present?*

A: A U.S. citizen must present a passport when entering or departing the United States by air. If traveling by land or sea, any proof of U.S. citizenship that clearly establishes identity and nationality is permitted, such as a birth record or baptismal record, along with government-issued photo ID, such as a driver's license.

An alien who is a lawful permanent resident of the United States must present a Permanent Resident Card ("Green Card," Form I-551), a Reentry Permit, or a Returning Resident Visa. For further information, see "How Do I Become a Lawful Permanent Resident While in the United States?" and "How Do I Get a Travel Document?"

Q: *How Can I Appeal?*

A: In certain circumstances, if you used a valid visa to apply for admission and your application for admission has been denied, you can request a hearing before the Immigration Court, where an immigration judge will determine your case. A judge's decision can be appealed to the Board of Immigration Appeals (BIA). You will receive instructions on where and how to appeal. If you apply for admission to the United States under the Visa Waiver Pilot Program, the decision of the officer is final. In cases involving fraud, willful misrepresentation, false claim to U.S. citizenship or lack of a valid immigrant visa for an intending immigrant, the officer's decision is final.

Appendix C:
Migration Resources

In This Appendix

International Council of Nurses Position Statement on the Ethical Recruitment of Nurses

Migration Correspondence Tracking Form

U.S. Licensure Fees Tracking Form

INTERNATIONAL COUNCIL OF NURSES POSITION STATEMENT ON THE ETHICAL RECRUITMENT OF NURSES

Ethical Nurse Recruitment

ICN Position

ICN and its member associations firmly believe that quality health care is directly dependent on an adequate supply of qualified and committed nursing personnel, and support the evidence that links good working conditions with quality service provision. ICN recognises the right of individual nurses to migrate,[1] and confirms the potential beneficial outcomes of multicultural practice and learning opportunities supported by migration. The Council acknowledges the adverse effect that international migration may have on health care quality in countries seriously depleted of their nursing workforce.

---

[1] There is the basic assumption that the recruited persons have the qualifications and experience required to meet the criteria imposed by the regulatory body of the recruiting country/province/state to practice as a nurse

ICN condemns the practice of recruiting nurses to countries where authorities have failed to implement sound human resource planning and to seriously address problems which cause nurses to leave the profession and discourage them from returning to nursing.

ICN denounces unethical recruitment practices that exploit nurses or mislead them into accepting job responsibilities and working conditions that are incompatible with their qualifications, skills and experience.

ICN recognises the benefits of circular migration and calls for mechanisms to support nurses who wish to return to their home countries.

ICN and its member national nurses associations call for a regulated recruitment process based on ethical principles that guide informed decision-making and reinforce sound employment policies on the part of governments, employers and nurses, thus supporting fair and cost-effective recruitment and retention practices.

These key principles include:

Effective human resources planning, management and development, leading to national self-sustainability: Effective planning and development strategies must be introduced, regularly reviewed and maintained to ensure a balance between the supply and demand of nurse human resources. While it is essential that local and national planning, management and development lead to the self-sustainability of national health workforces, globalisation will increasingly highlight the importance of human resources planning and development at the international level. An essential dimension of human resources development is continuing education. Nurses must be ensured access to programmes that will maintain their competence and support their advancement as health professionals while maintaining a high level of knowledge, skill and commitment for the provision of quality care.

Credible nursing regulation: Nursing legislation must authorise the regulatory body to determine nurses' standards of education, competencies and standards of practice. Regulatory bodies must ensure that only individuals meeting these standards are allowed to practise as a nurse.

Access to full employment: The provision of quality care relies on the availability of nurses to meet staffing demand. Nurses in a recruiting region/country and seeking employment should be made aware of job opportunities. If necessary, health stakeholders (especially government and employers) need to explore policies that would facilitate nurses' active participation in the workforce such as family-friendly environments and reinsertion programmes.

Freedom of movement: Nurses have the right to migrate if they comply with the recruiting country's immigration/work policies (e.g. work permit) and meet obligations in their home country (e.g. bonding responsibilities, tax payment). Faced with a growing multicultural patient population, establishing a multicultural provider workforce supports culture-sensitive health care provision.

Freedom from discrimination: Nurses have the right to expect fair treatment such as working conditions, promotion, and continuing education. (*Note*: Cases of positive discrimination need to be considered separately.)

Good faith contracting: Nurses and employers are to be protected from false information, withholding relevant information, misleading claims and exploitation (e.g. accurate job descriptions, benefits/allocations/bonuses specified in writing, authentic educational records). Access to factual employment-related information must be guaranteed, including social or daily life information (e.g. access to accommodation, compassionate leave, sick leave). The concept of informed consent must be applied to all parties involved in employment contract negotiation.

Equal pay for work of equal value: There should be no discrimination between occupations/professions with the same level of responsibility, educational qualification, work experience, skill requirement, and hardship (e.g. pay, grading). Similarly there must be no discrimination between persons within the same profession with the same level of responsibility, educational qualification, experience, skill requirement, and hardship.

Access to grievance procedures: When nurses' or employers' contracted or acquired rights or benefits are threatened or violated, suitable machinery must be in place to hear grievances in a timely manner and at reasonable cost.

Safe work environment: Nurses must be protected from occupational injury and health hazards, including violence (e.g. sexual harassment) and made aware of existing workplace hazards. Effective prevention, monitoring, and reporting mechanisms must be in place. Protocols for withdrawal of services in situations of life-threatening danger to the nurse need to be established.

Effective orientation/mentoring/supervision: The provision of quality care in the current highly complex and often stressful health care environment depends on a supportive formal and informal supervisory infrastructure. Nurses have the right to expect proper orientation and on-going constructive supervision within the work environment.

Employment trial periods: Employment contracts must specify a trial period when the signing parties are free to express dissatisfaction and cancel the contract with no penalty. In the case of international migration, the responsibility for covering the cost of repatriation needs to be clearly stated.

Freedom of association: Nurses have the right to affiliate to and be represented by a professional association and/or union in order to safeguard their rights as health professionals and workers. Partnerships between the associations/unions in the recruiting and recruited countries could facilitate the exchange of timely and accurate information. They would also ensure the continuation of a supportive professional environment providing needed assistance.

Regulation of recruitment: Recruitment agencies (public and private) should be regulated and effective monitoring mechanisms introduced (e.g. cost-effectiveness, volume, success rate over time, retention rates, equalities criteria, client satisfaction). Disciplinary measures must be introduced sanctioning agencies whose practice is unethical.

These principles are the foundation for ethical recruitment whether international or intra-national contexts are being considered. The recruitment and retention of nurses has become an urgent priority and a growing expense. All health sector stakeholders—patients, governments, employers and nurses—will benefit if this ethical recruitment framework is systematically applied.

Nurses need to be well-informed. National nurses associations have a responsibility to provide information and lobby for the elimination of abusive recruitment practices.

Background

Career mobility is important both to nurses in furthering their careers and to society in allowing nursing to adapt and respond to changing health needs. Career mobility enables nurses to achieve personal career goals and contributes to the nursing profession by raising the competency of its members. It allows nursing to respond to scientific, technological, social, political and economic changes by modifying or expanding the roles, composition and supply of nursing personnel to meet identified health needs.

A complex web of contributing factors generates the global nursing workforce imbalances (see "Recruitment/Retention Crisis Factors"). The current situation, characterised by an increasing demand and a decreasing supply, results in heightened competition for the nursing human resources available, both within and among countries. Countries or health care facilities have come to regard international migration as a permanent although partial solution to their nursing shortage. Examples are not limited to the industrialised countries but also include recruitment among developing countries even within the same geographic region (e.g. Caribbean, Southern Africa). Moreover, this trend is not restricted to registered professionals but also applies to students at the basic and post-basic level.

Many internationally recruited nurses report that they would prefer to remain in their home country, with their family and friends in a familiar culture and environment. The quality of work life in many countries needs to be improved before migration will significantly decrease. Before resorting to aggressive recruitment campaigns, government and employers faced with the challenges of a shortage need to address the contributing factors relevant to their situation. Aggressively recruiting nurses or students into a dysfunctional health/ nursing system is neither cost-effective nor ethical. The goal is to have self-sustainable national nursing workforces, which acknowledge the contribution of international professionals yet guarantee a stable core of care providers to meet health needs.

In some cases, unscrupulous recruitment agents take advantage of uninformed nurses. In response to chronic (often cyclical) nursing shortages world-wide, national health services or independent care organisations have negotiated the recruitment of nurses among their own nationals and/or foreign nurses. Private for-profit agencies have increasingly become involved in the search for nursing personnel. Recently, aggressive international recruitment is on the increase. This type of recruitment focuses on large numbers of recruits, sometimes significantly depleting a given health facility or contracting an important number of newly graduated nurses from a given educational institute. There is usually no designated body that regulates or monitors the content of contracts offered. Nurses may be employed under false pretences or misled as to the conditions of work and possible remuneration and benefits. Internationally recruited nurses may be particularly at risk of exploitation or abuse; the difficulty of verifying the terms of employment being greater due to distance, language barriers, cost, etc.

Increasingly there have been calls for an ethical framework for nurse recruitment. The principles supporting such a framework are relevant to international as well as intra-national recruitment. Their credibility, strength and universality will directly depend on the political will of health sector stakeholders and the regulatory mechanisms introduced for their application and monitoring.

Recruitment/Retention Crisis Factors

Increased Demand	■ Reduced lengths of stay in hospital (generated by advanced technology and new financing systems) increasing the acuity of care
	■ Shift from hospital to ambulatory, home and community care creating a fast growing labour market for nurses outside hospital facilities
	■ Ageing population emphasising long-term health care services, multi-system involvement, and increased acuity
	■ Recent increase in number of nursing education places and programmes requiring greater numbers of faculty
	■ Increased number of specialties
	■ Growing private sector expanding the labour market
	■ Globalisation expanding the labour market
	■ Greater nurse entrepreneurship opportunities expanding the labour market
	■ Nurse considered by the public as a professional worthy of trust and chosen as the primary entry point to health services
	Increased opportunities and demand for nurses outside the nursing service (e.g. generic management).
Decreased Supply	■ Reduced student pool (i.e. general education level)
	■ Increased career opportunities for women
	■ Ageing nursing workforce (e.g. retirement, lighter workloads desired)

(Continued)

Recruitment/Retention Crisis Factors (Continued)
<ul><li>Ageing nursing faculty</li><li>Increasing number of mature students with reduced potential years of professional practice</li><li>Decreased funding of nursing schools and heavier financial burden on students</li><li>Past government decisions to reduce nursing student positions</li><li>Reduced number of nurses interested in academic careers and teaching positions</li><li>Increased family career obligations (e.g. care of an elderly parent).</li><li>Poor working conditions, including pay</li><li>Increased career opportunities outside the health care sector, including better pay and working conditions</li><li>Lack of accommodation, transport</li><li>Occupational health hazards</li><li>Nurse burnout</li><li>Inadequate support staff</li><li>Poor image of the profession as a career.</li></ul>

Adopted in 2001

Revised and reaffirmed in 2007

MIGRATION CORRESPONDENCE TRACKING FORM

Make a copy of this page or write directly on this page to keep up with the U.S. visa and licensure process.

Document or Information Sent	Where Sent	Date Requested and Date Mailed	Notes

U.S. LICENSURE FEES TRACKING FORM

The U.S. licensure process for a foreign-educated nurse can involve a number of fees. These can be paid directly to the organizations by the nurse if you choose to do so and need not be paid through a third party. The following checklist will assist you in compiling a list of fees for the state in which you are seeking licensure. You can make a copy of this to record what you will need to pay for and what you have already paid for. Check with the particular State Board of Nursing where you are seeking licensure to determine which services are required and what the fees are.

Cost in U.S. Dollars	Service or Application
	Test of English Language Proficiency
	Certification Program Certificate
	VisaScreen Certificate
	Board of Nursing application fee for licensure by examination
	NCLEX-RN or NCLEX-PN application fee
	International testing fee (if taking NCLEX-RN or NCLEX-PN examination outside of the United States or its territories)
	Board of Nursing temporary permit fee
	Credentials evaluation fee
	Fingerprinting service
	Transcripts from school of nursing program
	Other
	Other
	TOTAL

Appendix D:
CGFNS International Reports

In This Appendix

Sample CGFNS Certification Program Pass Letter

Sample Certification Program Fail Letter

Explanation of Client Need Categories

Sample Nursing and Science CES Report

Sample Full Education CES Report

SAMPLE CGFNS CERTIFICATION PROGRAM PASS LETTER

CGFNS INTERNATIONAL

3600 Market Street, Suite 400, Philadelphia, Pennsylvania 19104-2651 U.S.A. Applicant Inquiries: 215.349.8767 • Automated Phone System: 215.599.6200 • Web: www.cgfns.org

December 10, 2008
CGFNS #

PASSED

Dear Ms.

The Commission on Graduates of Foreign Nursing Schools (CGFNS) is pleased to report that you achieved a passing score on the 11/12/2008 CGFNS Qualifying Exam. The passing score for each examination is set at 400. Your score on the 11/12/2008 examination was: 460.

Listed below are the Client Need Categories (in bold) and subcategories that form the basis of not only the CGFNS Qualifying Exam, but also the NCLEX-RN Examination. The 'X' in each box shows your performance in the categories. A description of each Client Need Category and the content included is provided on the back of this letter. Since the CGFNS Qualifying Exam is a predictor of performance on the NCLEX-RN Examination, knowledge of your performance in these categories will help you to prepare for that examination. If your performance (denoted by the 'X') is outside the shaded area in any Client Need Category, your preparation for the NCLEX-RN® Examination should focus on that category.

Congratulations on your successful completion of the CGFNS Qualifying Exam.

Performance Level		
	Poorer	Better
Safe Effective Care Environment	X	
Management of Care	X	
Safety and Infection Control		
Health Promotion and Maintenance		X
Psychosocial Integrity	X	
Physiological Integrity		X
Basic Care and Comfort	X	
Pharmacological and Parenteral Therapy		X
Reduction of Risk Potential	X	
Physiologic Adaptation		X

SAMPLE CGFNS CERTIFICATION PROGRAM FAIL LETTER

CGFNS INTERNATIONAL
3600 Market Street, Suite 400, Philadelphia, Pennsylvania 19104-2651 U.S.A. Applicant Inquiries: 215.349.8767 • Automated Phone System: 215.599.6200 • Web: www.cgfns.org

December 10, 2009
CGFNS #

FAILED

Dear Ms.

On 11/12/2008 you sat for the CGFNS Qualifying Exam. Unfortunately, you did not achieve a passing score on the examination. The passing score for each examination is 400. Your score on the 11/12/2008 examination was: 298.

Listed below are the Client Need Categories (in bold) and subcategories that form the basis of not only the CGFNS Qualifying Exam, but also the NCLEX-RN Examination. The 'X' in each box shows your performance in the categories. A description of each Client Need Category and the content included is provided on the back of this letter. Since the CGFNS Qualifying Exam is a predictor of performance on the NCLEX-RN Examination, knowledge of your performance in these categories will help you to prepare for that examination. If your performance (denoted by the 'X') is outside the shaded area in any Client Need Category, your preparation for retaking the CGFNS Qualifying Exam should focus on that category.

Performance Level		
	Poorer	**Better**
Safe Effective Care Environment	X	
Management of Care	X	
Safety and Infection Control	X	
Health Promotion and Maintenance	X	
Psychosocial Integrity	X	
Physiological Integrity	X	
Basic Care and Comfort		X
Pharmacological and Parenteral Therapy	X	
Reduction of Risk Potential	X	
Physiologic Adaptation	X	

EXPLANATION OF CLIENT NEED CATEGORIES

The four Client Needs categories included in the CGFNS and NCLEX-RN® Test Plans are: Safe, Effective Care Environment, Health Promotion and Maintenance, Psychosocial Integrity and

Physiological Integrity. Below are descriptions of the areas of nursing covered by each category.

A. Safe, Effective Care Environment

Management of Care: providing integrated, cost-effective care to clients by coordinating, supervising and/or collaborating with members of the multidisciplinary health care team. Specific areas of knowledge include, but are not limited to, advance directives, advocacy, case management, client rights, concepts of management, confidentiality, continuity of care, continuous quality improvement, delegation, ethical practice, incident/irregular occurrence/variance reports, informed consent, legal responsibilities, organ donation, consultation and referrals, resource management, and supervision.

Safety and Infection Control: protecting clients and health care personnel from environmental hazards. Specific areas of knowledge include, but are not limited to, accident prevention, disaster planning, error prevention, handling hazardous and infectious materials, medical and surgical asepsis, standard (universal) precautions, other precautions, and use of restraints.

B. Health Promotion and Maintenance

Assisting clients and their significant others through the normal, expected stages of growth and development from conception through advanced old age. Specific areas of knowledge include, but are not limited to, aging process, ante/intra/postpartum and newborn developmental stages and transitions, expected body image changes, family planning, family systems, and human sexuality. Also includes managing and providing care for clients in need of prevention and early detection of health problems. Specific areas of knowledge include, but are not limited to, disease prevention, health and wellness, health promotion programs, health screening, immunizations, lifestyle choices, and techniques of physical assessment.

C. Psychosocial Integrity

Promoting client ability to cope, adapt and/or problem solve situations related to illnesses or stressful events. Specific areas of knowledge include, but are not limited to, coping mechanisms, counseling techniques, grief and loss, mental health concepts, religious and spiritual influences on health, sensory/perceptual alterations, situational role changes, stress management, support systems, and unexpected body image changes. Also includes managing and providing care for clients with acute or chronic mental illnesses. Specific areas of knowledge include, but are not limited to, behavioral interventions, chemical dependency, child abuse/neglect, crisis intervention, domestic violence, elder abuse/neglect, psychopathology, sexual abuse, and therapeutic milieu.

D. Physiological Integrity

Basic Care and Comfort: providing comfort and assistance in the performance of activities of daily living. Specific areas of knowledge include, but are not limited to, assistive devices, elimination, mobility/immobility, non-pharmacological comfort interventions, nutritional and oral hydration, personal hygiene, and rest and sleep.

Pharmacological and Parenteral Therapies: managing and providing care related to the administration of medications and parenteral therapies. Specific areas of knowledge include, but are not limited to, administration of blood and blood products, central venous access devices, chemotherapy, expected effects, intravenous therapy, medication administration, parenteral fluids, pharmacological agents and actions, side effects, total parenteral nutrition, and untoward effects.

Reduction of Risk Potential: reducing the likelihood that clients will develop complications or health problems related to existing conditions, treatments, or procedures. Specific areas of knowledge include, but are not limited to, alterations in body systems, diagnostic tests, lab values, pathophysiology, potential complications of diagnostic tests, procedures, surgery and health alterations, and therapeutic procedures.

Physiologic Adaptation: managing and providing care to clients with acute, chronic or life-threatening physical health conditions. Specific areas of knowledge include, but are not limited to, alterations in body systems, fluid and electrolyte imbalances, hemo dynamics, infectious diseases, medical emergencies, pathophysiology, radiation therapy, respiratory care, and unexpected response to therapies.

SAMPLE NURSING AND SCIENCE CES REPORT

Credential Evaluation Service (CES)
Nursing and Science Course-by-Course Report

Prepared For: IL DEPT OF PROF
                              REGULATION/CONTINENTAL
                              TESTING SRV
                              DIVISION OF PROFESSIONAL
                              REGULATION
                              320 WEST WASHINGTON,
                              3RD FL SPRINGFIELD,
                              ILLINOIS 62786
                              UNITED STATES OF AMERICA

Applicant Name: MARY SAMPLE

Other Name:

CGFNS ID Number: 0000000

Social Security Number: NONE

Mailing Address: 1234 ANY STREET
                              APT 3B.
                              ANY CITY, PENNSYLVANIA 12340

Birth Date: June 19, 1985

Country of Nursing Ed: PHILIPPINES

Dates of Attendance: June 2003–March 2007

CGFNS Certificate Status: Not a CGFNS Certificate Holder as
                              of this review

Purpose of Report: Licensure

MARY SAMPLE
CGFNS ID # 0000000
Part I: Page 2 of 7

Non-Nursing Education

CGFNS has evaluated the following non-nursing education credential(s).

I. Credential Name: Secondary School Diploma

Name of Institution: GENERAL SANTOS HOPE CHRISTIAN SCHOOL

Address of Institution: General Santos City, Philippines

Completion Date: March 2007

Source of Credential: Applicant

Explanation:

- **Entrance Requirement:** Completion of six years of primary school education

- **Length of Study:** Four years for a total of ten years of primary and secondary school education

- **Nature of Study:** General

- **Gives Access To:** Philippines' National College Entrance Examination (NCEE). Sufficient scores on the NCEE give access to freshman admission to a college or university in the Philippines. May be considered for freshman admission to most colleges and universities in the United States with an NCEE score in the 75th percentile or if grades are superior. Students with insufficient academic grades and NCEE scores below the 75th percentile may be required to complete grade 11 or 12, or pass the examination for General Educational Development to be admitted to some colleges and universities in the United States depending on admission standards

■ **Comparability:**   Comparable to the completion of high school in the United States

Comments: The secondary school diploma is the terminal credential for secondary education in the Philippines. It is awarded after completion of ten years of primary and secondary school education. No NCEE score was indicated on the applicant's academic record.

Nursing Education

CGFNS has evaluated the following Nursing education credential(s).

I. Credential Name: Official Academic Transcript for a Bachelor of Science in Nursing Program

Name of Institution: SAN PEDRO COLLEGE

Address of Institution: DAVAO CITY, Philippines

Government Approved: YES

MARY SAMPLE
CGFNS ID # 0000000
Part I: Page 4 of 7

Dates of Attendance: June 2003–March 2007

Completion Date: March 2007

Source of Credential: School

Explanation:

- **Entrance Requirement:**   Successful completion of ten years of primary and secondary school education and sufficient scores on the Philippines' National College Entrance Examination or the equivalent

- **Length of Study:**   Four years

- **Nature of Study:**   General nursing

- **Language of Instruction:**   English with English textbooks.

- **Gives Access To:**   Nursing licensure examination and advanced nursing education in the Philippines. May be considered for graduate admission to most colleges and universities in the United States. Students whose academic record and test scores are not adequate for graduate admission in the United States may be considered for undergraduate admission with transfer credit determined on a course-by-course basis or for provisional graduate status.

■ **Comparable To:**   Comparable to a Bachelor of Science in Nursing program in the United States.

Comments: This credential, however, represents completion of only ten years of primary and secondary school education followed by four years of university for a total of fourteen years of education

Professional License/Registration

CGFNS has evaluated the following professional license/registration credential(s).

I. Credential Name: Validation of Registration for a Registered Nurse

Registration Number: 000000

Issuing Agency: PROFESSIONAL REGULATION COMMISSION

Address of Agency: P.O. BOX 2038 MANILA, 1008, Philippines

Date of Issue: May 10, 2008

Expiration Date: See Comments

Validation Date: September 12, 2008

Source of Credential: PROFESSIONAL REGULATION COMMISSION

Professional Title: Registered Nurse

MARY SAMPLE
CGFNS ID # 0000000
Part I: Page 6 of 7

Explanation

- **Education Requirements:** Completion of a first-level general nursing program at a government-approved school of nursing and passing the Philippines nurse licensing examination

- **Scope of Practice:** Provide nursing care and supervision of patients of all ages in hospital or community settings; observe and accurately report facts and evaluations; supervise other personnel contributing to the nursing care of patients

- **Gives Access To:** Employment as a registered nurse in the Philippines

- **Comparable To:** Comparable to the registration of a first-level general (registered) nurse in the United States.

Comments: The Professional Regulation Commission has indicated to CGFNS that renewal of professional licenses is no longer mandatory in the Philippines. The applicant's license has never been disciplined and is valid until revoked. This information was current as of September 12, 2008.

Note: This report reflects the general comparability of foreign credentials to US credentials, and is not intended to denote exact equivalence. The evaluations contained herein are based on the standards approved by the National Council on the Evaluation of Foreign Educational Credentials and other information sources as noted. Unless otherwise stated, all transcripts used in this evaluation were received directly from the source. This report is advisory in nature, and is intended to provide guidelines and recommendations. It is not intended as a substitute for the autonomous evaluation and decision-making of an organization.

EVALUATOR: Mary Jones   **DATE: October 16, 2008**

Report recipient inquiries: 215/222-8454
Applicant Inquiries: 215/349-8767

(Monday–Thursday, 9:00 A.M.–5:00 P.M., Eastern Time)
(Friday, 9:00 A.M.–4:30 P.M., Eastern Time)

SAMPLE FULL EDUCATION CES REPORT

Credential Evaluation Service (CES)
Course-by-Course Report

Prepared For:

UNIVERSITY OF PENNSYLVANIA
3400 SPRUCE STREET
PHILADELPHIA,
PENNSYLVANIA 19104
UNITED STATES OF AMERICA

Applicant Name: Mary Sample

CGFNS ID Number: 0000000

Mailing Address: 2345 ANY STREET
ANY TOWN,
PENNSYLVANIA 12345
USA

Social Security Number: NONE

Birth Date: December 13, 1966

Country of Nursing Ed: PHILIPPINES

Dates of Attendance: June 1986–April 1989

CGFNS Certificate Status: Not a CGFNS Certificate Holder as
of this review

Purpose of Report: Employment

Non-Nursing Education

CGFNS has evaluated the following non-nursing education
credential(s).

I. Credential Name: Secondary School Diploma (Katunayan)

Name of Institution: Juan Sumulong Memorial Junior College

Address of Institution: Taytay, Rizal, Philippines

Completion Date: March 1981

Source of Credential: Applicant

Explanation:

- **Entrance Requirement:** Completion of six years of primary school education

- **Length of Study:** Four years for a total of ten years of primary and secondary school education

- **Nature of Study:** General

- **Gives Access To:** Philippines' National College Entrance Examination (NCEE). Sufficient scores on the NCEE give access to freshman admission to a college or university in the Philippines. May be considered for freshman admission to most colleges and universities in the United States with an NCEE score in the 75th percentile or if grades are superior. Students with insufficient academic grades and NCEE scores below the 75th percentile may be required to complete grade

11 or 12 or pass the examination for General Educational Development to be admitted to some colleges and universities in the United States depending on admission standards.

■ **Comparable To:** Comparable to the completion of high school in the United States.

Comments: The secondary school diploma is the terminal credential for secondary education in the Philippines. It is awarded after completion of ten years of primary and secondary school education. The applicant attained an NCEE score in the 88th percentile.

Nursing Education

CGFNS has evaluated the following Nursing education credential(s).

I. Credential Name: Official Academic Transcript for a Bachelor of Science in Nursing Program

Name of Institution: QUEZON CITY MEDICAL CENTER & COLLEGES (AKA WORLD CITI COLLEGES)

Address of Institution: QUEZON CITY, Philippines

Government Approved: YES

MARY SAMPLE
CGFNS ID # 0000000
Part II: Page 4 of 14

Dates of Attendance: June 1987–April 1990

Completion Date: April 1990

Source of Credential: School

Explanation:

■ **Entrance Requirement:** Successful completion of ten years of primary and secondary school education and sufficient scores on the Philippines' National College Entrance Examination or the equivalent

■ **Length of Study:** Four years

■ **Nature of Study:** General nursing

■ **Language of Instruction:** English with English textbooks

■ **Gives Access To:** Nursing licensure examination and advanced nursing education in the Philippines. May be considered for graduate admission to most colleges and universities in the United States. Students whose academic record and test scores are not adequate for graduate admission in the United States may be considered for undergraduate admission with transfer credit determined on a course-by-course basis or for provisional graduate status.

- **Comparable To:**   Comparable to a Bachelor of Science in Nursing program in the United States.

Comments: This credential, however, represents completion of only ten years of primary and secondary school education followed by four years of university for a total of fourteen years of education. According to an analysis of the academic record, this program was 57 percent nursing coursework and 43 percent science and humanities coursework. (This breakdown is calculated based solely on coursework completed in the Bachelor of Science in Nursing program.)

Professional License/Registration

CGFNS has evaluated the following professional license/registration credential(s).

I. Credential Name: Validation of Registration for a Registered Nurse

Registration Number: 0000000

Issuing Agency: PROFESSIONAL REGULATION COMMISSION

Expiration Date: See Comments

Validation Date: November 20, 2007

Source of Credential: PROFESSIONAL REGULATION
COMMISSION

Professional Title: Registered Nurse

Explanation:

■ **Education Requirement:**   Completion of a first-level general nursing program at a government-approved school of nursing and passing the Philippines nurse licensing examination

■ **Scope of Practice:**   Provide nursing care and supervision of patients of all ages in hospital or community settings; observe and accurately report facts and evaluations; supervise other personnel contributing to the nursing care of patients

■ **Gives Access To:**   Employment as a registered nurse in the Philippines.

■ **Comparable To:**   Comparable to the registration of a first-level general (registered) nurse in the United States.

Comments: The Professional Regulation Commission has indicated to CGFNS that renewal of professional licenses is no longer mandatory in the Philippines. The applicant's license has never been disciplined and is valid until revoked. This information was current as of November 20, 2007.

MARY SAMPLE
CGFNS ID # 0000000
Part II: Page 7 of 14

II. Credential Name: Validation of Registration for a Registered Nurse (Part 1)

Registration Number: 00000000

Issuing Agency: NURSING & MIDWIFERY COUNCIL

Address of Agency: 23 PORTLAND PLACE LONDON, W1B 1PZ, United Kingdom

Date of Issue: October 28, 2002

Expiration Date: October 30, 2005

Validation Date: September 20, 2007

Source of Credential: NURSING & MIDWIFERY COUNCIL

Professional Title: Registered Nurse (Part 1)

Explanation:

- **Education Requirements:** Completion of a first-level general nursing program at a government-approved school of nursing and passing the United Kingdom Central Council licensure examination for general nurses administered by the United Kingdom Central Council for Nursing, Midwifery and Health Visiting (UKCC).

- **Scope of Practice:** Conduct and carry out a comprehensive assessment and plan of nursing care; work with and/or manage a team of nurses, medical and para-medical personnel, and social worker

- **Gives Access To:**   Employment as a registered general nurse (Part 1) in the United Kingdom.

- **Comparable To:**   Comparable to the license of a first-level general (Registered) nurse in the United States

Comments: The Statement of Entry documents initial entry in the Professional Register of the United Kingdom Central Council for Nursing, Midwifery and Health Visiting (UKCC). Current licensure/registration is documented by the nurse's Personal Identification Card issued by the UKCC. The applicant's license has never been disciplined or revoked. This information was current as of September 20, 2007. Re-registration is required.

III. Credential Name: Validation of Registration and Examination Scores for a Registered Nurse

Registration Number: 0000000

Issuing Agency: COLLEGE OF NURSES OF ONTARIO

Address of Agency: 101 Davenport Rd.

Toronto, Ontario, M5R 3P1 Canada

Date of Issue: September 22, 2004

MARY SAMPLE
CGFNS ID # 0000000
Part II: Page 9 of 14

Expiration Date:	December 31, 2008
Validation Date:	December 27, 2007
Source of Credential:	COLLEGE OF NURSES OF ONTARIO
Professional Title:	Registered Nurse

Explanation:

- **Education Requirements:** Completion of a first-level general nursing program and passing the Canadian Nurses Association Testing Service (CNATS) Comprehensive Examination for Nurse Registration/Licensure

- **Scope of Practice:** Apply professional nursing knowledge or service for the purpose of assisting a person to achieve and maintain optimal health through promotion, maintenance and restoration of health, or prevention of illness, injury or disability; care for the sick and dying; provide health teaching and counseling; coordinate health care

- **Gives Access To:** Employment as a registered nurse in Ontario, Canada.

- **Comparable To:** Comparable to the registration of a first-level general

(Registered) nurse in the United States.

Quezon City Medical Center & Colleges (AKA World Citi Colleges)

Dates of Attendance: June 1986 to April 1989

	Transcript Hours	Transcript Grade	Comparable U.S. Credit	U.S. Grade Hours
1986				
Nursing Courses				
Nsg. Care Mgmt. 101: Foundation of Nursing Practice I w/Related Learning Experience	6	2.00	4.50	B
Nsg. Care Mgmt. 102: Foundation of Nursing Practice III w/Related Learning Experience	9	1.60	6.75	A–
Teaching Strategies	3	2.10	2.25	B
Other Courses				
Essay Writing	3	1.90	2.25	B
Physical Education III	1	1.90	0.75	B
Physical Education IV	1	1.80	0.75	B+
Rizal Course	3	1.70	2.25	B+
Science Courses				
Anatomy and Physiology	5	1.60	3.75	A–
Micro/Parasitology	4	2.20	3.00	B–
Nutrition	3	2.80	2.25	C
1987				
Nursing Courses				
Nsg. Care Mgmt. 103: Nursing Practice I w/Related Learning Experience	11	2.00	8.25	B
Nsg. Care Mgmt. 104: Nursing Practice II w/Related Learning Experience	13	2.10	9.75	B

(Continued)

	Transcript Hours	Transcript Grade	Comparable U.S. Credit	U.S. Grade Hours
Other Courses				
Advanced Spanish	3	2.00	2.25	B
Agrarian Reform and Taxation	3	1.75	2.25	B+
Economics	3	1.60	2.25	A–
Speech and Oral Communication	3	2.00	2.25	B
Science Courses				
College Algebra	3	1.70	2.25	B+
General Physics	3	2.40	2.25	C+
Political Science	3	1.90	2.25	B
1988				
Nursing Courses				
Elective Nursing Practice	3	2.00	2.25	B
Nursing Courses				
Health Ethics	3	1.80	2.25	B+
Nsg. Care Mgmt. 105: Nursing Practice III w/Related Learning Experience	9	2.25	6.75	B–
Nsg. Care Mgmt. 106: Nursing Practice IV w/Related Learn. Exp.	10	2.25	7.50	B–
Other Courses				
Asian Civilization	3	2.60	2.25	C+
Moral, Social and Civic Education	–	Passed		–
Philippine Literature in Spanish	3	2.00	2.25	B
Science Courses				
Computer and Society	3	2.00	2.25	B
Socio-Anthropology	3	2.00	2.25	B

MARY SAMPLE
CGFNS ID # 0000000
Part II: Page 13 of 14

Comments: Additional information received by CGFNS from QUE-
ZON CITY MEDICAL CENTER & COLLEGES (AKA WORLD
CITI COLLEGES) on December 7, 2006, indicated that the applicant received the following hours of theoretical instruction and hours
of clinical practice:

Area of Nursing	Theory	Clinical
Care of the Adult-Medical	126	260
Care of the Adult-Surgical	144	284
Maternal/Infant	108	284
Care of Children	108	284
Psychiatric/Mental Health	90	162

Trinity College of Quezon City

Dates of Attendance: June 1985 to March 1986

	Transcript Grade	Transcript Hours	Comparable Grade	U.S. Credit
1985 **Nursing Courses**				
Elementary Spanish	3	1.75	2.25	B+
Intermediate Spanish	3	2.25	2.25	B–
Introduction to Humanities	3	2.5	2.25	C+
Introduction to Literature	3	2.0	2.25	B
Life & Works of Jesus	–	1.25		
Logic	3	2.00	2.25	B

(Continued)

	Transcript Grade	Transcript Hours	Comparable Grade	U.S. Credit
Panitikang Pilipino	3	2.25	2.25	B–
Personalities of the Old Testament	–	1.75		B+
Philippine History	3	2.25	2.25	B–
Sining ng Pakikipagtalastasan	3	1.75	2.25	B+
Science Courses				
College Algebra	–	–		
Elementary Biochemistry	5	3.0	3.75	C
General Chemistry	5	3.0	3.75	C
General Zoology	5	2.75	3.75	C
Introductory Psychology Adesola Adegbite	3	1.5	2.25	A–

This report reflects the general comparability of foreign credentials to US credentials, and is not intended to denote exact equivalence. The evaluations contained herein are based on the standards approved by the National Council on the Evaluation of Foreign Educational Credentials and other information sources as noted. Unless otherwise stated, all transcripts used in this evaluation were received directly from the source. This report is advisory in nature, and is intended to provide guidelines and recommendations. It is not intended as a substitute for the autonomous evaluation and decision-making of an organization.

EVALUATOR: Mary James   **DATE: October 16, 2007**

Report recipient inquiries: 215/222-8454
Applicant Inquiries: 215/349-8767

(Monday–Thursday, 9:00 A.M.–5:00 P.M., Eastern Time)
(Friday, 9:00 A.M.–4:30 P.M., Eastern Time)

Appendix E: Slang Terms, Idioms, Jargon, and Abbreviations

In This Appendix:

Slang Terms, Idioms, and Jargon for Living in the United States

Slang Terms, Idioms, and Jargon Commonly Heard in Nursing Practice Situations

List of Common Abbreviations Heard in Nursing Practice Situations

SLANG TERMS, IDIOMS, AND JARGON FOR LIVING IN THE UNITED STATES

Slang Term or Idiom	*Actual Meaning*
"All in all…"	Taking everything into consideration. For example, "All in all, it was a good day."
ASAP	As soon as possible
"He/she has an attitude problem."	Phrase used to describe someone who is antagonistic or argumentative.
"I'm having a bad hair day."	Phrase used to describe a day in which nothing seems to go right or the way you planned it.
Bye-bye	Shortened form of saying good-bye.
"I'm just chilling."	Phrase to describe a period when you are relaxing so that you don't feel stressed.

Slang Term or Idiom	Actual Meaning
"Everything's cool."	Term used to mean that everything is all right.
"Correct!"	Term used to assure another that he/she understands what you have said. For example, the other person says, "so, you've completed all your work." Your response might be, "Correct" instead of "Yes."
"I have to do the dishes."	Phrase indicating the need to wash and dry the dishes used during a meal.
"He/she is driving me nuts."	Phrase used to describe someone whose behavior is bothering you.
"I'm fixing to…"	"I plan to…"
"From now on"	From this moment forward.
FYI	For your information
"How you doing?"	Term used to ask another person how they are.
"Later."	Term used to close a conversation—meaning that the person will see you or talk to you at another time.
"Make up your mind."	Phrase used when telling someone to make a decision.
Messed up	Can be used to describe a mistake, e.g., "I messed up," or to describe a person who is having difficulty managing his/her life, e.g., "He's messed up."
"Never mind!"	Phrase used to tell someone not to do something you previously requested, e.g., "Never mind doing that assessment." Can also be used in a negative sense or tone when you become frustrated when another individual does not seem to understand what you are asking or saying, e.g., "Oh, never mind!"

Slang Term or Idiom	*Actual Meaning*
Off the hook	Phrase used to describe no longer being required to do something or to be accountable for something, e.g., "I'm off the hook for that error."
Pocket book	A purse or handbag
Pop, soda, and Coke	Three terms used to mean essentially the same thing—soda pop
Quarter of 8	Used as an expression of time, i.e., 7:45
"I'm screwed."	I'm in trouble
"Sorry? "	Way of asking someone to repeat what he/she said
STAT	Immediately
"Take it easy."	Term used to end an interaction—used instead of good-bye. Can also be used to try to calm someone down.
"What've you been up to?"	Form of greeting that doesn't require full disclosure of all activities in which you are involved. Usually a short answer, such as "I've been working a lot of hours at the hospital" will suffice.
"What's up?"	Term used as a form of greeting, instead of hello. Does not require a lengthy explanation of what you have been doing. A simple response such as "Not much" or "I'm excited about starting work" followed by asking about the other person will suffice.
"Y'all"	Contraction for you all. Used when conversing with a group of people. For example, "How y'all doing?" Used more frequently in the southern part of the United States.

SLANG TERMS, IDIOMS, AND JARGON COMMONLY HEARD IN NURSING PRACTICE SITUATIONS

Slang Term or Idiom	*Actual Meaning*
"I'll give him a piece of my mind"	To give another your opinion, usually in anger.
Badge	Identification card
"I can't seem to get my wind"	Indicates that the person is short of breath
Code blue; Call a code	General terms used to indicate the need to mobilize the emergency team (physician, anesthesiologist or anesthetist, nurses, and other health care personnel) when a patient experiences cardiac arrest, respiratory arrest, or life-threatening cardiac arrhythmias.
Come down with	Phrase used to describe becoming ill, e.g., "I seem to be coming down with a cold."
"I can't seem to come out of it."	Can't seem to move on with one's life after an illness or depression.
"Will you crank up my bed?"	Term used to mean raise the head of the bed.
"I'm under the weather."	Term used to mean that the person is feeling ill.
Goof off	Term used to describe not working or doing something else when one should be working, e.g., "He's goofing off."
"He's a pain in the neck."	Phrase used to describe someone who annoys you.
"I'm tied up right now."	I don't have time to help you
"I need to have a BM."	I need to make a bowel movement
"We need to run fluids."	Need to give intravenous fluids to rehydrate a patient.

Slang Term or Idiom	*Actual Meaning*
"I need to do number 1."	"I need to urinate."
"I need to do number 2."	"I need to move my bowels."
"She's out to lunch."	Phrase describing someone who is oblivious to what is happening.
The patient passed or passed away	The patient has died.
"Do you have to pee?"	Slang way of asking if a person has to urinate.
Do you need to use the restroom?	Refers to using the toilet or bathroom.
"I'm going to throw up."	"I'm going to vomit."
"It really tickled my fancy."	Something that appealed to you, e.g., "Seeing him really tickled my fancy."
"What's cooking?"	Form of greeting asking about what is going on in your life. Similar to "What's happening?"
"I'll push it through."	Making sure that what you are requesting is done, e.g., "I'll push through your request for additional staff."
Yo!	Form of greeting comparable to saying hello.

LIST OF COMMON ABBREVIATIONS HEARD IN NURSING PRACTICE SITUATIONS

Abbreviation	*Meaning*
ABD	Type of abdominal pad or dressing
ABGs	Arterial blood gasses
ABT	Antibiotic therapy
ac	Before meals
AMA	Against medical advice
APAP	Automatic Positive Airway Pressure. An APAP machine automatically adjusts on a breath by breath basis to deliver the minimum pressure needed to keep an airway open while asleep.
ARDS	Acute respiratory distress syndrome
ASAP	As soon as possible
bid	Twice a day
bpm	Beats per minute
CA	Cancer
CABG	Coronary Artery Bypass Graft
CAD	Coronary Artery Disease
CCU	Critical Care Unit
CHF	Congestive Heart Failure
COPD	Chronic obstructive pulmonary disease
CPAP	Continuous Positive Airway Pressure (CPAP)— a common treatment for obstructive sleep apnea. CPAP is produced by a machine that delivers pressurized air to a nasal mask. This airflow acts like a splint to the airway, keeping it open and enabling uninterrupted sleep.
C-section	Cesarean section
CSF	Cerebral spinal fluid

Abbreviation	*Meaning*
CVA	Cerebral vascular accident
Detox	Detoxification
dig	Digoxin
DNR	Do not resuscitate
DOA	Dead on arrival
DOB	Date of birth
Drsg	Dressing
DSD	Dry sterile dressing
Dx	diagnosis
ER	Emergency room or department
Foley	Foley catheter; a type of indwelling, urethral catheter
FYI	For your information
GERD	Gastroesophageal Reflux Disease
GVHD	Graft versus Host Disease—seen following organ transplantation; usually indicative of organ rejection
Hep-C	Hepatitis C
hoh	Hard of hearing
hs	Hour of sleep
Hx	history
I&O	Intake and output
IV	intravenous
IVPB	IV piggyback; secondary intravenous connected to primary tubing
K	Potassium
KCl	Potassium chloride
KUB	An examination of the kidneys, ureters, and bladder

Abbreviation	Meaning
KVO	Keep vein open; Intravenous fluids are run at a slow rate so that the vein is preserved for subsequent IVs.
Labs	Laboratory values
LOC	Level of consciousness
Lytes	Electrolytes
MOM	Milk of Magnesia—a laxative
MRSA	Methicillin resistant staphylococcus aureus
MS	Multiple Sclerosis
MVA	Motor vehicle accident
NANDA	North American Nursing Diagnosis Association
NIDDM	Non-insulin Dependent Diabetes Mellitus; Type 2 Diabetes
Nitro	Nitroglycerin
NKA	No known allergies
NPO	Nothing by mouth
NSAID	Non-steroidal anti-inflammatory drugs; Used to relieve pain and inflammation
NVD	Nausea, vomiting and diarrhea
OB	Obstetrics
od	once daily
OOB	Out of bed
os	Left eye
ou	Both eyes
PCA	Patient controlled anesthesia
PD	Peritoneal dialysis
PEEP	Positive End Expiratory Pressure; Parameter used as a measure of maintaining acceptable gas exchange and to minimize adverse effects in patients on ventilators

Abbreviation	*Meaning*
PICC	Peripherally inserted central catheter; used for long-term, intravenous administration of drugs, such as antibiotics
Pit	Pitocin
po	By mouth
prn	As needed
ptca	Percutaneous Transluminal Coronary Angioplasty; procedure used when coronary arteries are blocked.
ROM	Range of motion
stat	Right away/immediately
tid	Three times a day
Vanco	Vancomycin—an antibiotic
Vent	Ventilator
VS	Vital Signs

Note: The Joint Commission has attempted to limit the use of abbreviations in health care settings. This list was identified by foreign nurse graduates as abbreviations they had seen on patient charts and could not understand. The editors of this book do not suggest that you use these abbreviations in your practice.

Appendix F: Educational Resources

In This Appendix

Select Listing of Schools for Online Nursing Degrees

SELECT LISTING OF SCHOOLS FOR ONLINE NURSING DEGREES

Benedictine University Online (www.onlinedegrees-benedictine.com)

Master of Science in Nursing

Capella University (www.capella.edu)

PhD in Nursing Education

Florida Hospital College of Health Sciences (www.onlineimaging.fhchs.edu)

Nursing (RN-to-BSN)

Gonzaga University (www.gonzagaonline.com)

MS in Nursing—Health Systems Leadership
MS in Nursing—Nurse Educator

Grand Canyon University (www.online.gcu.edu)

Nursing (RN-to-Bachelor's)
Nursing Education (Master's)

Nursing Leadership (MBA/Master's)
Nursing Leadership in Healthcare (Master's)

**Jacksonville University
(www.jacksonvilleeu.com/online-nursing-degree.asp)**

Nursing/Health Care Education (Master's)
Nursing/Healthcare Management (MBA)

Kaplan University Online (www.online.kaplanuniversity)

Nursing (RN-to-BSN)
Nursing/Nurse Administrator (Master's)
Nursing/Nurse Educator (Master's)

Saint Xavier University (www.sxuonline.com)

Clinical Nurse Leader (Master's)

South University (www.online.southuniversity.edu)

Nursing (RN-to-BSN)
Nursing (Master's)

**Stevens-Henager College Online
(www.elearners.com/college/stevens-henager-college/)**

Nursing Administration (Bachelor's)
Nursing Administration (Master's)

University of Cincinnati (www.uc.edu/distance/)

Nurse Midwifery (Master's)
Women's Health Nurse Practitioner (Master's)

**University of Phoenix (www.phoenix.edu/online_and_
campus_programs/online_and_campus_programs.aspx)**

Nursing/Health Care Education (Certificate)
RN-to-BSN (Bachelor's)
Nursing (Master's)
Nursing and Health Administration (Master's)

**University of Saint Mary
(www.stmary.edu/online/default.asp)**

Nursing—RN-to-BSN (Bachelor's)

Walden University Online (www.waldenu.edu)

Bachelor of Science in Nursing (BSN)

M.S. degree in Nursing (RN—MS degree program in Nursing—Education)

M.S. degree in Nursing (RN—MS degree program in Nursing—Leadership & Management)

M.S. degree in Nursing (RN)—MS degree program in Nursing—Informatics)

M.S. degree program in Nursing (BSN—MS degree program in Nursing—Education)

M.S. degree program in Nursing (BSN—MS degree program in Nursing—Informatics)

Glossary

Acculturation program: A system of procedures or activities that has the specific purpose of training individuals to understand another culture and its practices.

Accreditation: Type of quality assurance process under which services and operations of an institution or program are evaluated by an external body to determine if applicable standards are met. Should standards be met, accredited status is granted by the external body.

Adjudicate: To settle a case by lawful procedure.

Advanced practice nurses (APNs): Registered nurses who are educated at the master's level; have advanced theory and clinical education, knowledge, skills, and scope of practice; and can practice as independent practitioners. Includes nurse practitioners, clinical nurse specialists, certified nurse anesthetists, and certified nurse midwives.

Advocacy: Active support for a cause or position.

Affidavit: A sworn statement or written declaration made in the presence of someone authorized to administer pledges.

Alternative therapies: Therapeutic or preventive health care practices, such as homeopathy, naturopathy, chiropractic, and herbal medicine, that complement conventional medical methods.

Apprenticeship: Where one works with a skilled professional as a trainee.

Assertiveness: Ability to state one's position positively and in a self-confident manner.

Associate degree: A degree earned on completion of a 2-year program of study at a community college, junior college, technical school, or other institution of higher education.

Asylum status: Protection and immunity from extradition granted by a government to a foreign political refugee.

Attestation: The action of stating that something is true, especially in a formal written statement.

Auditing: The process of reviewing, evaluating, and verifying accounts or documents, especially those of a business, organization, or institution.

Automated Teller Machines (ATMs): Street-side computerized devices that provide bank customers with access to their accounts and the ability to withdraw money from remote locations.

Backlog: A quantity of unfinished business or work that has built up over a period of time and must be dealt with before progress can be made.

Biomedical research: Medical research and evaluation of new treatments for both safety and efficacy in what are termed clinical trials, and all other research that contributes to the development of new treatments.

Bioterrorism: Terrorism by intentional release or dissemination of biological agents, for example, bacteria, viruses, or toxins.

Botanicals: Drugs or products made directly from plants.

Breach of contract: A legal concept in which a binding agreement is *not* honored by one or more of the participants.

Centers for Medicare and Medicaid Services (CMS): The federal agency responsible for administering the Medicare, Medicaid, SCHIP (State Children's Health Insurance), HIPAA (Health Insurance Portability and Accountability Act), and CLIA (Clinical Laboratory Improvement Amendments) programs and several other health-related programs. Formerly known as the Health Care Financing Administration (HCFA).

Certification: Reflects achievement beyond the basic level of nursing and possession of expert knowledge in a particular area of practice.

Check card purchase: Buying an item that reduces the balance in your bank account using a bank debit card.

Codes of Conduct: Sets of rules outlining the responsibilities of, or proper practices for, individuals or the members of an organization or profession.

Codified: Signifies that laws have been collected and arranged in a systematic order.

Collective bargaining: Negotiations between management and a union about pay and conditions of employment on behalf of all the workers in the union.

Community-based care: Services provided in one's own home or other community settings; a variety of health care options that allow people to stay in their homes, while still providing important health care support.

Compliance: Readiness to conform or agree to do something; a state in which someone or something is in accordance with established guidelines, specifications, or legislation.

Congruence: Internal and external consistency; conformity or agreement.

Consular: Having to do with a consul, an official appointed by the government to reside in a foreign country to represent the commercial interests of foreign citizens who come from the official's home country.

Continuing education: Regular courses or training designed to bring professionals up to date with the latest developments in their particular field.

Coordinated care: Includes strategies to make health care systems more cost-effective and responsive to the needs of people with complex chronic illnesses.

Credentials evaluation: An analysis of an individual's qualifications, for example, education and licensure documents, to ensure that they are comparable to U.S. qualifications.

Credit history: Record of an individual's past borrowing and repayment of money. Includes history of late payment and bankruptcy.

Credit rating: An estimate of somebody's ability to repay money given on credit based on credit history.

Credit union: Owned and controlled by its members, a cooperative bank association that provides loans and other financial services to its members.

Criminal background check: The investigation of or search for the possibility of a person's criminal history; generally used by potential employers, lenders, and so forth, to assess the person's trustworthiness.

Cross-cultural communication: Interaction between two or more individuals of different cultures.

Cultural competence: An ability to interact effectively with people of different cultures.

Cultural conflicts: Disagreements that arise due to misunderstandings in communication and personal interpretations of words and actions.

Curative care: Refers to treatment and therapies provided to a patient with intent to improve symptoms and cure the patient's medical problem.

Debit card: A plastic card that provides an alternative payment method to cash when making purchases; also known as a bank card *or* check card.

Default clause: Section in a document; part of a contract that explains the consequences if someone fails to pay a debt or to meet a financial obligation.

Department of Homeland Security (DHS): A U.S. government agency created in 2003 to handle immigration and other security-related matters. A component of DHS is the Citizenship and Immigration Services, the government agency that oversees lawful immigration to the United States.

Department of Labor (DOL): The federal department responsible for improving working conditions and promoting opportunities for profitable employment in the United States.

Department of State: The U.S. government department that sets and maintains foreign policies, runs consular offices abroad, and makes decisions about nonimmigrant visas and immigrant visas that are processed through U.S. consulates.

Diagnostic report: Detailed information used to identify or reflect the results of a test.

Direct deposit: Electronic delivery of a paycheck directly into an individual's bank account by the individual's employer.

Disaster preparedness: Process of ensuring that an organization is prepared in the event of a forecasted disaster to minimize loss of life, injury, and damage to property and can provide rescue, relief, rehabilitation, and other services after the disaster.

Educational comparability: Where instructional coursework under one educational system is mostly equivalent to that of another.

Electronic transfer: Computer-based system used to perform financial transactions electronically.

Endorsement: Acceptance by one U.S. state of a professional license issued to an individual by another U.S. state or jurisdiction.

Ethnocentrism: Belief in the superiority of one's own ethnic group.

Extended care facilities: A medical institution that provides prolonged care (as in cases of prolonged illness or rehabilitation from acute illness).

Focus group: A small group of people who are questioned about their opinions as part of research.

Garnished wages: Monies taken from payroll or royalty checks, or from investment checks, to pay a debt.

Homeless shelter: Last resort in temporary housing for people in need who do not have a place to live.

Hospice: A usually small residential institution for terminally ill patients where treatment focuses on the patient's well-being rather than a cure and includes drugs for pain management and often spiritual counseling.

Human resource department: Section of an organization responsible for coordinating the recruitment and hiring of employees as well as maintaining the organization's implementation of labor laws.

Identity theft: Theft of personal information, such as someone's bank account or credit card details.

Idiom: An expression of speech whose meaning is translated figuratively rather than literally.

International Council of Nurses (ICN): A federation of 128 national nurses associations that focuses on the education, practice, and economic and general welfare of nurses worldwide.

Internship: Where one works as a trainee gaining practical, on-the-job experience for a specified amount of time, for example, as a new nurse graduate in a hospital critical care unit.

Jargon: A form of language used by people who work together within a specific occupation or profession or within a common interest group.

The Joint Commission: Independent, nonprofit organization that evaluates and accredits more than 15,000 health care organizations and programs in the United States; the nation's predominant standards-setting and accrediting body in health care.

Labor certification: Process of proving that an employer has ensured that there are no qualified U.S. workers for the position being offered to a foreign worker.

Learner-focused: Education focused on the learner's needs and their learning styles.

Licensed practical nurse: A technical nurse with 12–18 months of training who has passed the state licensure examination for practical nurses (NCLEX-PN) and who works under the supervision of a registered nurse.

Mandatory overtime: Where employers *require* employees to work more than the standard 40 hours per week.

Meals on Wheels: Provides home-delivered meals to people in need, usually the elderly or the disabled.

Mentor: A senior or experienced person in a company or organization who gives guidance and training to a junior colleague; a wise and trusted teacher and counselor.

Municipal hospitals: Hospitals controlled by city government.

North American Free Trade Agreement (NAFTA): A trade agreement that allows for the exchange of products and services in North America, involving the United States, Canada, and Mexico.

Notarized signature: A notary's stamp and signature that signifies that something, such as a signature on a legal document, is authentic and legitimate.

Nurse Practice Act: Group of laws governing nursing practice.

Nursing process: A step-by-step, problem-solving approach that includes assessment, analysis or diagnosis, planning, implementation, and evaluation.

Palliative care: A specialized form of care focused on the pain, symptoms, and stress of serious illness.

Patient self-care: Type of care in which the patient assumes accountability for health care and participates in the planning of that care.

Peer review: An assessment of an article, piece of work, or research by experts on the subject.

Pen pal: Two people, usually in different countries, who become friends through an exchange of letters but who may never meet.

Petition: An appeal to or request made of a higher authority.

Portfolio: A collection of items or documents outlining one's work experience, achievements, and skills organized in a binder, file, or electronic format.

Preceptor: A specialist in a profession, especially health care, who gives practical training to a student or novice in the profession.

Prevailing wage: Defined as the hourly wage, usual benefits, and overtime paid in the largest city in each county to the majority of workers.

Professional autonomy: Responsible discretionary decision making by a profession or an individual within the profession; the quality or condition of being self-governing.

Public policy expert: An individual who has studied and/or works in the branch of political science that deals with the formation of laws or policies.

Refugee status: Protection granted by a government to someone who has fled another country, often because of political oppression or persecution.

Registered nurse: A professional nurse with 2–4 years of education who has passed the state licensure examination for registered nurses (NCLEX-RN).

Regulatory authority: A public authority or government agency responsible for enforcing standards and safety, overseeing the use of public goods and services, as well as regulating commerce; also, the power to control or direct an entity in agreement with a law or regulation.

Remittance: The portion of migrant income that, in the form of either funds or goods, goes back into the home country.

Residency programs: Positions wherein one works for a specific period of time in a community or a facility to gain experience. In many U.S. facilities such programs are structured learning experiences.

Retribution: Something meted out or given to someone as punishment for something he or she has done.

Retrogression: The procedural delay in issuing an immigrant visa when there are more people applying for immigrant visas in a given year than the total number of visas available.

Role-playing: Practicing how you will respond in a situation by playing the part you will take or that of another person, for example, practicing your interaction with a physician who has written an order that you must question.

Scam: A scheme for making money by dishonest means.

Scope of practice: Refers to what a professional is legally authorized to do.

Security deposit: A sum of money required by somebody selling something or leasing property as security against the buyer's or tenant's failure to fulfill the contract.

Self-learning modules: Activities designed for participants to undertake independently when they are unable to attend traditional education sessions.

Shared governance: A set of practices under which management and staff join in decision making.

Slang: Highly informal words or expressions that are not considered standard in the language.

Specialty certification: Validation of competence, recognition of excellence, or legal regulation in a specialty area of practice.

Telenursing: Refers to the use of information technology for providing nursing services in health care.

Test of nursing knowledge: An examination that tests understanding of the major areas of nursing (adult health nursing, nursing of children, maternal/infant nursing, and psychiatric/mental health nursing), critical thinking ability, and ability to apply nursing principles to the clinical situation.

Third-party authorization: Occurs when the individual for whose benefit a contract is created gives another person the right to act on that individual's behalf.

Translational scientists: Scholars who integrate research inputs from the basic sciences, social sciences, and political sciences to optimize both patient care and also preventive measures that may go beyond the provision of health care services.

Tuition reimbursement: Employer payment for a course of study. The employer may pay for the course before it starts or pay back course fees paid by the employee after completion of the course and attainment of a passing grade.

Unencumbered: Not held back or delayed because of difficulties or problems, for example, a nursing license that is not revoked, suspended, or made probationary or conditional by a licensing or regulatory authority as a result of disciplinary action.

Union: An organization of workers who have banded together to achieve common goals in key areas such as wages, hours, and working conditions.

U.S. Citizenship and Immigration Service (USCIS): The U.S. government agency that oversees lawful immigration to the United States. It establishes immigration services, policies, and priorities and adjudicates the petitions and applications of potential immigrants.

Video conference: Live audio and visual transmission of meeting activities to bring people at different sites together.

Vocational nurse: A graduate of an accredited technical school of nursing; licensed practical nurses (LPNs) are known as licensed vocational nurses (LVNs) in California and Texas.

Voluntary overtime: Where an employee offers or agrees to work for pay in excess of the standard 40 hours per week.

Index